Slimming with

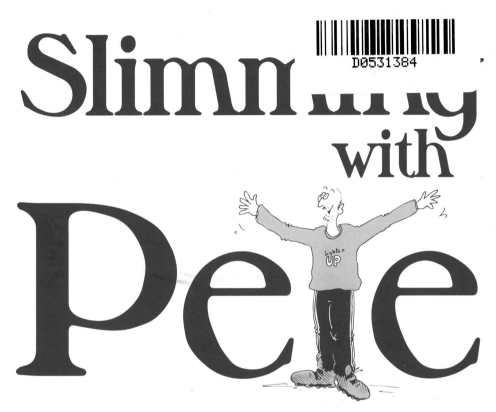

Taking The Weight Off Body AND Mind

Pete Cohen & Judith Verity

Crown House Publishing Limited
www.crownhouse.co.uk

First published in the UK by

Crown House Publishing
Crown Buildings
Bancyfelin
Carmarthen
Wales
www.crownhouse.co.uk

First published 1998; reprinted 1998, 1999, 2000

British Library of Cataloguing-in-Publication Data
A catalogue entry for this book is available
from the British Library.

ISBN 1899836136

Printed and bound in Wales by

Hackman Print Group

*The characters in this book are fictional. Any resemblance to any individual,
whether living or dead, is purely coincidental.*

Introduction

Dedication

This book is dedicated to the hundreds of slimmers and exercisers
I have worked with over the years, including those whose stories
inspired the book.

Acknowledgements

To Andy Sellins for your encouragement, support and friendship always.

To Madeleine Cotter for your early input and advice.

To Colin & Shellie Deans for your work on the weight management programme and your input to this book.

To Andy Blackburn for your time and dedication in illustrating my ideas and drawing me.

To Michele Humphrey for all the love and support you gave me.

To Helene Hilltout and Sandy Stuckey for your feedback and encouragement.

To Richard Bandler and John Grinder, the originators of NLP (Neuro-Linguistic Programming), and other contributors to this field, some of whose techniques and ideas have been utilised in this book.

To Paul McKenna, thank you for your kind words and support.

To Mitch and Tina Davis. Without you, none of this would have been possible.

And to my Mum and Dad, Judith and David Cohen, for all your support and endless encouragement. Thank you.

About The Authors

Pete Cohen

Pete Cohen has worked in the Health and Fitness industry for twelve years as a sports psychologist, personal trainer and lecturer in sports science and nutrition, and he is well known for his work with teams and individuals. He is currently working as sports psychologist and motivator to Kent County Cricket club and the British Blind Cricket Team as well as with a number of well-known athletes.

Seven years ago, Pete developed the Lighten Up weight control method using sports psychology techniques, NLP, and much of his own insight and wisdom. Lighten Up has proved hugely successful and his audiotape and this first book, *Slimming With Pete*, have become hugely popular.

Unlike many other slimming gurus, Pete doesn't have a weight problem himself. But, if you ask him whether he really understands the desperation of people caught in the dieting trap, he will tell you he has plenty of experience in overcoming problems and succeeding in the face of enormous difficulties. Diagnosed severely dyslexic as a child and told that further education would be out of the question, he now has more degrees than GCSEs as well as a bestselling book to his name. Pete Cohen is one of those people who never gives up on a problem until he finds the solution.

His warmth, energy and enthusiasm have made him hugely popular on TV and in the media, but he is a natural entertainer and teacher and, for him, there is no substitute for working directly with the people he is helping. So, his work as a sports psychologist continues and he still runs his inspirational Lighten Up workshops and eight-week evening courses. Although he isn't able to do as many of these as he would like, there is a weekend workshop every month and a new evening course every ten weeks.

Working with Pete is always a memorable and life-enhancing experience.

Judith Verity

Judith Verity has twenty-eight years of varied experience as a probation officer, counsellor, trainer, businesswoman and writer. In the 1980s she ran her own training and office management company, eventually selling out in order to concentrate on teaching and writing. She has a particular interest in dieting problems and has worked with people suffering from eating disorders. When she met Pete Cohen and he told her his story, she was so inspired by it that they decided to work together to put Lighten Up into writing. To date they have written two books together, this one and *Doing it with Pete, The Lighten Up Slimming Fun Book.*

Introduction

This book is about the people I work with and the methods I use to help them out of the dieting trap. I know that dieting is a huge and partly hidden problem. I've met people who have spent thirty years of their lives dieting, and more. And they still haven't lost weight. I've met bright, beautiful people like Lisa who were putting more effort into watching their weight than living their lives. Some of them were even risking their health in the process.

Then there are people like Mo, who get caught up in the image process almost accidentally, only to find it invades their privacy and grows like a parasite out of control. And so many others squeeze a hectic working schedule or a demanding family into a day with too few hours, leaving no time or energy for keeping fit and enjoying sensual pleasures to the full, eating being just one of those.

As a health and fitness professional and nutritionist, I know how to look after my body. As a person, I want to have fun. I've learned that the key to being the shape you want is putting those two together. And I know that the one sure way to gain weight and give yourself pain and grief at the same time is to focus on your personal larder. If, while you're doing this, you happen to be relying on a diet as well, then you're really in a mess. A diet, a set of rules, a routine, a regime, a calorie counter and a can of artificial milk shake isn't going to help you. It's going to make you feel more out of control. And that's the scary thing about being overweight. It's not until you take back the control and responsibility for yourself and get to know yourself better that you'll start to see changes.

If you've tried to lose weight in the past and haven't succeeded, would you say it was because you haven't been good enough at any of these:

Getting It Right, Trying Hard, Having Enough Willpower, Being Disciplined, Working At It, Concentrating, Being Determined, Being Motivated Enough...?

If you decide to read this book, remember, forget all of the above. This is just a bit of fun.

If you would like to use the ideas and techniques in this book, contact us at Lighten Up on 020 8241 2323 or visit our website: lightenup.co.uk. There are one day workshops and a few eight-week evening courses you might like to join and the detailed, step-by-step guide to the Lighten Up Programme is now available in ***Doing it with Pete, the Lighten Up Slimming Fun Book.*** Pete has also made a tape which talks you through some of his key exercises.

Chapter One

A Diet To Die For

On the way to the club one Saturday morning I called in on Mo and Lisa. The sandwich shop was closed on Saturdays, and their kitchen was always good for breakfast and a chat. Lisa answered the door; even at ten o'clock on a weekend she looked elegant, if a little dissipated. Her blond hair was scraped back from her face but she'd already got her eye make-up on. Either that or she hadn't taken it off from the night before. I followed her into the kitchen. There was a smell of toast and stale beer. Mugs, plates and crumbs seemed to be everywhere.

'Hi Pete.' Mo didn't even look up from the newspaper. 'Did you know that diets can kill you?' She was getting butter and croissant crumbs all over the crossword.

'Don't I know it.' Lisa was back to measuring out two cups of unsweetened muesli and half a cup of skimmed milk. 'I probably won't have time for lunch,' she said, 'I think I'll have my two pieces of fruit now with breakfast.'

'You can't,' Mo reminded her. 'You finished off the bananas last night when we got in from the pub, said you needed something to soak up the booze.'

'Oh God, no wonder my head hurts,' said Lisa, pulling a bottle of Nurofen out of the microwave.

'Anyway,' Mo waved the paper at her, 'according to this article, traditional diets – which one are you on now, by the way? – are very bad for the health.'

'Is that mental health?' I wondered, as I put some bread under the grill.

'No, I'm serious, you can get so obsessed with losing weight that you don't eat properly.'

I turned to look at her. 'My idea of a diet is at least three meals a day.'

'Pete' said Lisa, 'there are times when you can be really annoying.'

'How many diets have you been on?' I asked her.

'Just count the books up there on the shelf. Actually I've done some of them twice, plus I've got some tapes in the car...'

I looked at the dresser. There were as many diet books as cookery books, and a lot of them had pictures on them of slender, glowing people, dressed in colourful, figure-hugging lycra. I suppose the implication was that if you read the book and stuck to

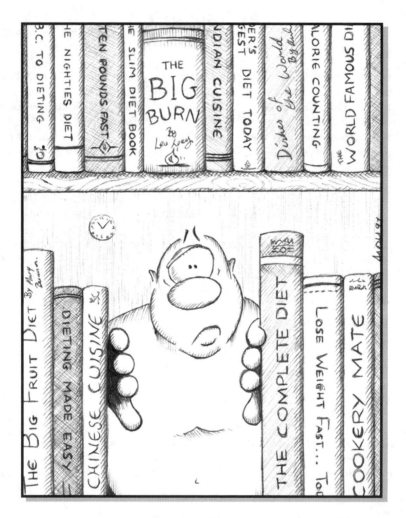

Living With the Enemy

the diet, you would look like the picture on the cover. One of them, by a famous chat show host even had a banner headline saying "Lose 10 pounds in 10 days". I grabbed it off the shelf and waved it at Lisa.

'If you believe that you'll believe anything – nobody can lose more than two pounds of fat in a week,' I said.

Mo looked up, 'Surely he couldn't say he did if he didn't? Not that I care; he looks just as sleazy in the "after" photos as he did in the "before" photos.'

'He might have lost 10lb, but it wouldn't be ten pounds of fat and there's no point in losing anything else.' I held up the book again, 'Can I borrow this by the way?'

Lisa squinted at it. 'I haven't got my lenses in yet… oh, that one. You're welcome to it, that diet never did anything for me - I lost the weight but, as soon as the diet finished, it went straight back on. What's more, I gained it back even faster than I lost it!'

Diets have been happening all around me ever since I can remember and I never took any notice. I assumed that dieting was one of those facts of life which wouldn't affect me – like clothes and periods. I didn't find out until much later how mistaken I was about that.

My mother was on a diet, and so were my friends' mothers and sisters; but, as far as I knew, our fathers and brothers weren't. Since my Mum never got any thinner, I asked her once why she bothered with diets when they didn't make any difference. 'They do make a difference' she said, 'but it doesn't last.'

'Why not?'

'Because you can't stay on a diet forever.'

When I was a teenager I noticed that my girlfriends often ate most of my chips, but they never bought any of their own. It wasn't that they were mean – they didn't mind paying for cinema tickets. Another interesting thing about girlfriends at that stage in my life was that they always knew how many calories there were in a Quarter Pounder in spite of the fact that they'd never have eaten one in a million years.

After that breakfast with Lisa and Mo, I started to think very hard about the whole dieting business. After all, it was a pretty major factor in my working life as well as a big preoccupation with a lot of my friends. When I thought about it, more than half the people who came to the club seemed more concerned with weight loss than anything else. I decided that maybe I should give it a bit more priority.

A week later, I went for a Lads' Night Out with some friends to a Mexican restaurant. One of the guys admired the menu and then ordered a salad – which he pushed around the bowl while we all ate.

'Ben, what the hell is the matter with you? Last time we came here we both had fajitas and I remember you finished mine as well as yours.'

For many dieters, every minute of the day is a potential mealtime

Food is always on their minds

'I'll be eating when I get home.'

'Gone off Mexican?'

'No, no, it's good, it's very good. But I just started with this food combining diet, you have to be careful what you eat with what ... it's just easier to do it yourself ...'

Suddenly he had everybody's attention. He's a bit older than the rest of us, an ex-rugby player who's teaching now at the local boy's school. He looks, well, just like you'd expect an ex-rugby back to look. Big, solid and tough. I remembered him from years ago when he was thinner and always seemed to get the attention of the girls I was interested in. Even now, he normally ate like he was still in training, though I have to admit, the curry and lager diet was really beginning to show up on his waistline. He was the last person I would ever have expected to eat a salad at a men's night out, and we gave him hell for letting the side down.

'What is it, Benjamin? The new girlfriend wants a thinner model?'

'He's been going to the Ladies Aerobics and his leotard doesn't fit ...'

Then, surprisingly, a couple of the others stood up for him. They'd heard of the diet and one of them had a friend who'd lost weight with it. We spent the rest of the evening talking about eating instead of sharing jokes and enjoying the food. Ben left early, and it was a while before I saw him again.

It was all beginning to look like glimpses of the same iceberg. It struck me that maybe people were dropping out of the exercise programmes at the gym for the same reason they were dropping out of diets. It seems like most people talk about eating well and exercising regularly, but even when they start they don't keep it up. When you hear them talk about it, you realise why. Dieting and exercise mean pain and deprivation to most people. It's hard work, something you have to force yourself to do when you'd rather be lying on the sofa watching Friends and eating a pizza. Hunger, exhaustion and aching muscles are the expectation, ever since Jane Fonda urged everyone to "go for the burn" and assured us that without pain there wouldn't be any gain. I always thought she really must have meant loss, but I suppose it doesn't rhyme. No wonder people give up and write themselves off, over and over again.

Once I started to focus on the problem, I suddenly started seeing diets everywhere. They were even making me feel uncomfortable. It's like buying a car. As soon as you get a new one, you realise that nearly everybody else has the same model and wonder why you never noticed it before.

Sometimes I felt like an alien. Why wasn't I planning my next meal as soon as I finished the last one and craving Mars bars in between? That's the way everybody else seemed to be operating. People on diets can make you feel weird for eating a chocolate biscuit, or a banana, or an avocado pear. You don't find out till later that they are actually eating the same things. It's just that they don't necessarily do it at mealtimes. For dieters it seems like every minute of the day is a potential mealtime. Food is always on their minds.

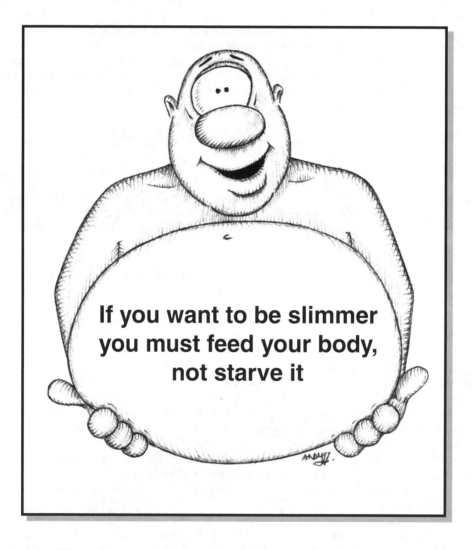

I don't think about food that often, but when I do get hungry I start thinking about what would taste good. I usually try out a few things in my mind before I decide what would feel best inside me. Eating is so much fun that there doesn't seem to be much point in wasting time on something you don't really, really want.

So I only really think about eating when I'm getting ready to eat. And I definitely didn't give much thought to not eating until one cold January Monday morning at the club. New Year is always tough because the customers feel guilty about all the partying and they're determined to pay for the fun they've had. I was running through the beginners' assessment with a middle aged banker whose latest wife had given him a year's membership for Christmas. I remember thinking "I wonder how long this marriage is going to last?" while I was chatting about his programme. Then I heard a thud behind me.

I looked around. My friend Lisa was lying on the floor. I'd persuaded her to start coming to the gym a couple of weeks earlier when we were having our usual conversation in her kitchen about losing weight. Or, as she saw it, not being able to lose enough weight.

By the time I got over to her she was already trying to get up again. I thought she'd be upset but I could see from her face that she wasn't worried, she was embarrassed. She wanted to get right back into her routine but Jane, one of the other trainers, put an arm round her and led her off to the cafe.

When I'd finished the banker's assessment I followed them. Lisa was sitting alone with a cup of coffee in one corner. She looked tired and transparent.

'What was that all about?' I asked her.

'Sorry Pete, it's this diet I started in the new year. I'm not allowed to eat anything before midday – maybe I'll change to the evening sessions until I'm at my target weight.'

'I thought the whole idea of coming here regularly was to get away from constantly dieting. I can remember you telling me and Mo last year that you were going to try a different approach to this weight problem you seem to think you've got. I thought you were happy with the way things were going. I think you look even thinner than you did when you were calorie counting all the time.'

'I'm still calorie counting. You can't give up dieting just like that. I've always had to watch what I eat. The exercising is an extra bit of help that's all – I let myself have a few treats the days I come to the club.'

All the time I was looking at her. It's funny how you get so used to people that you don't see them any more. Lisa's one of those cool blondes with the traditional look of deceptive fragility. At least, I used to think it was deceptive. As we sat in the cafe I noticed that she wasn't slender; she was thin. There's a difference – but I hadn't thought about it before.

'I'm getting quite interested in diets,' I told her, 'Tell me about it.'

If you always do
what you've
always done

You'll always get
what you've
always got

She was sipping her coffee and avoiding my eyes. 'Well, I've tried all sorts. I change diets fairly regularly ...'

'Why?'

'Oh, lots of reasons. I get bored. I can't stick to them and then I put back more weight than I lost. You name a diet and I bet I've been on it. In fact, just before Christmas I did go back to one that worked for me before. You know those slimming groups they run at the church hall? Well, that was a disaster. You won't believe this but the woman who runs it had a completely different system to the one she was running before. When we asked her why, she said "Oh, my ladies like a change". So I said to her "What you mean is, you've got the same bunch of fatties coming back over and over again and you've got to come up with something new because the previous permanent weight loss method you sold them only lasted six months!".'

'That sounds a bit harsh, what did she say to that?' I asked.

'She got really stroppy with me and said she thought it wouldn't be appropriate for me to rejoin the class because my negative attitude might de-motivate the other punters. "You mean you don't want them to spot the catch as well" I said. But, actually Pete, I had this nagging feeling that maybe she was right, maybe I do have a negative attitude that's causing me to fail all the time.'

I was as mad as she was by this time. 'You're not a failure,' I told her. 'The diets have all failed you. How long are you going to go on like this? Doesn't changing from one kind of eating pattern to another play havoc with your digestion?'

'Well, yes, it can be embarrassing occasionally. I had a pretty antisocial couple of weeks on the fibre diet.' She was smiling a bit now. 'But if you keep changing to a new diet routine, it's not so easy to cheat. It keeps you on your toes. I'm fine with my current one during the week, but it's really hard to stick to it at weekends. This Friday it was one of my colleagues' birthday so we went out for a drink and after a couple of hours in the pub I thought I might as well go for a curry with everybody else. Then on Saturday I met a girlfriend who's just split with her fiancé and there's nothing like a long lunch for talking somebody through a broken heart. It works brilliantly because it makes you feel good at the time and then afterwards the depression about eating and drinking too much overshadows losing the relationship. It's perfect.'

'Anyway,' she went on, 'after the lunch, I had a dinner date on the Saturday night and by Sunday I was feeling guilty. So I went for a run and stayed away from the fridge. I just stuck to apples and oranges and drank lots of water.'

'Did you have breakfast this morning?'

'No, didn't have time, I'll have something when I get to work. In theory I'm only supposed to eat fruit before midday but I usually have something a bit more substantial before I come to the club.'

'You know, it's a lot better to eat something before midday if you want to burn it off quickly.'

A DIET TO DIE FOR

Where there's a will, there's always a way

'Maybe,' she said, 'but once you start a diet you have to stick with the rules, otherwise the whole thing just doesn't work. Anyway, it's different for you, isn't it? You don't have to worry about your weight like the rest of us.'

'Suppose I could teach you how I do it – how I control my weight and stay fit, would that help?'

'Of course it would, but you couldn't, could you? People like you come from some planet where you can programme yourself to the size and shape you want and then forget about it. You're naturally thin, you've probably got thin parents, thin genes and a high metabolic rate. You can't teach people how to change the way they are inside. Anyway, fitness is the way you earn a living, the rest of us get paid for sitting in front of a VDU and talking down the telephone.'

That was the challenge that changed the way I worked for good and led me to set-up my first "Lighten Up" programmes. It took a while to work out the difference that made the difference between food-focused people and people who had figured out that there was more to life. Because diets are times of pain, denial and unhappiness, they tend to be temporary. So about 95 out of every 100 people on a diet will put back as many pounds as they lose and sometimes more. It's like betting on a horse that's got 5% chance of winning the race – I can't understand why so many people do it, but they do. I suppose they must be so desperate that 5% is better than no chance at all. Or perhaps they don't know the odds are so heavily stacked against them. £1 billion a year is spent on dieting and with currently half the male population and two out of every five women overweight in the UK alone (20 million overweight adults, 6 million classified as obese) the dieting industry looks set to boom even more.

Dieting affects the mind as well as the body. Deprived of our favourite foods we feel hungry and irritable. We disrupt our body's natural weight regulation system, making digestion difficult, and losing weight becomes even harder. There seems to be a tendency to revert to old eating patterns after a diet and the whole thing becomes something of a ritual, a constant cycle of new beginnings rather than a steady way of life.

Dieting can certainly be an addiction but the addiction isn't to the food, it's to dieting itself. After the incident at the club, I was worried about Lisa so I called in to see her later that week. She was looking better than she had on the Monday morning, and Mo, of course, was her usual cheerful self.

'Lisa told me about Monday' was the first thing she said to me when she answered the door. 'I just knew that would happen sooner or later. It's getting to be a pattern every bloody weekend now. She breaks the diet, she binges, then she starves herself to make up for it. And the worst of it is that we all have to suffer. She's so bad-tempered about the whole damn thing you wouldn't believe – and on top of that she goes around making us all feel guilty every time we have a biscuit.'

'Well, Lisa's always struck me as being a bit of a perfectionist' I said as we went down to the kitchen, 'in terms of appearances anyway. But it does sound like she's getting more extreme.'

The dieting industry makes vast sums of money out of failure

95 out of every 100 people who go on a diet put the weight back on when the diet finishes, yet in America the diet drinks industry is worth $16 billion, health clubs $9 billion and commercial weight loss programmes $2 billion.

'She's changed a lot. And, if you ask me, going to the gym first thing on Monday mornings is just one of the crazy things she does. The first day of the week's traumatic enough without making it worse – you wouldn't catch me doing it!'

'Is working out really that painful for you?' I was amazed. Myself, I get such a buzz from exercising that I can't really understand why people would bother to do it at all if it hurt.

Lisa was sitting in the kitchen and overheard me. She looked up, 'Pete, you are such a pain, exercising and dieting are not a normal human being's idea of a good time.'

'By "normal human beings" I suppose you mean women. So is it just men who enjoy working out?' I was trying to think whether I knew any men who were on diets. Before the girls had time to say anything I knew the answer. More and more of the men I knew who came to the club were calculating calories, worrying about the fat content of their sandwiches and desperately trying to get rid of their love handles.

'There are more overweight men than women' said Lisa.

Mo waved a dismissive hand. 'That's because the average man hasn't got the willpower to give up the beer and crisps.'

'If you're going to be sexist' I said. 'What scores higher in terms of human suffering – a man with a beer belly or a woman who can't enjoy a meal out with friends?'

It's really hard for me to accept that so many people could be prepared to disrupt their natural eating patterns to the point of making themselves ill just for the sake of a few pounds or inches. Especially since I know that we are eating 20% less food than we were 20 years ago. You'd think that eating less would mean more slender athletic people, but no, the average British adult has increased in weight by nine pounds over the last ten years and 47% of British women are size 16 or over.

Maybe it's just that we're evolving into different body sizes and shapes for some good reason. Now that so many jobs involve sitting in front of a computer we might as well turn into chair-shaped, pear-shaped blobs. Larger bums could be a considerable comfort factor for the future. Like built-in upholstery.

Or is the weight increase something to do with dieting?

Neither evolution nor dieting seems to be a very likely cause of weight gain, but let's take the dieting for a start.

Diets generally promote a drastic cut in the quantities of food consumed, sometimes even to the point of temporary starvation (look at poor Lisa in the gym that January morning; the spirit was willing, but the flesh was definitely weak). Unfortunately, the body is designed to ensure its owners survival under adverse conditions and adjusts its metabolic rate. It slows down drastically in response to a lower intake. This makes

Eating tends to be an automatic process,often done without much thought or appreciation

Get yourself a note pad and start writing down what you eat and drink.

Once you become aware of your habits and patterns, changing them becomes easier.

it difficult to digest what little food the diet allows. The body's next protecting move against starvation is to start storing the longest-lasting food source which of course is fat. In its attempt to save your life, your body is actually capable of burning lean muscle tissue to provide energy. It's like burning the furniture during a power failure.

Diets often don't promote a corresponding increase in energy consumption. The emphasis on calorie counting, weighing food portions and reading labels (not great calorie-burners compared to kneading dough or digging vegetables) tends to distract people from getting out and about, joining rumba classes and generally enjoying life.

So although the scales might look good after a week or so of cutting back on the wine and pizza, bear in mind that lean muscle tissue is three times as heavy as fat and, also, that less food tends to equal less water in the body as well. So you're kidding yourself. This is not the way to be healthy and slim and feel great. You really have to do yourself the favour of learning to trust your body and work with your own physiology instead of against it.

I know so many people who seem to think their body is some kind of enemy, working against them. Defeating them every time they want to buy a new outfit for a special date or feel good about themselves when they look in the mirror on Monday morning. Living with the enemy is no way to live. It's time to call a truce. Dieting is a waste of time. You can lose hours, days and weeks of your precious life on it and end up ill, depressed and, probably, fatter.

You may as well accept that it's time to turn around and make friends with yourself again. This book will help you find ways of doing just that.

You could begin just as soon as you've read the next few paragraphs. But before you start thinking about what changes you might make, I want you to know where this book came from and why it works. I first got involved in the problems of dieting and weight loss as a result of my work as a nutritional counsellor, personal trainer and sports psychologist. Throughout my professional career I've met hundreds of people who were suffering, really suffering; firstly because of a losing battle with their weight and secondly because of the useless, addictive and sometimes downright dangerous diets that were supposed to be helping them. Talk about a double whammy. I'm not saying that all diets are dangerous but some of the well known ones certainly are, and official statistics show that 95% of the time all of them certainly are useless.

The facts in this book (which are pretty simple and basic) are mainstream, current medical ones. You can trust them. I'm not offering you a magic formula, though there's plenty of magic in the book.

Even more important, I didn't just dream up the exercises by myself. This is probably a good time to say "thank you" to all the people I've worked with and learned from over the years. I may have put it all together, but I've learned how to make it work from the people whose battles I've been privileged to help fight. The weight control method in this book has been up and running now for five years and we have an amazing 80% success rate.

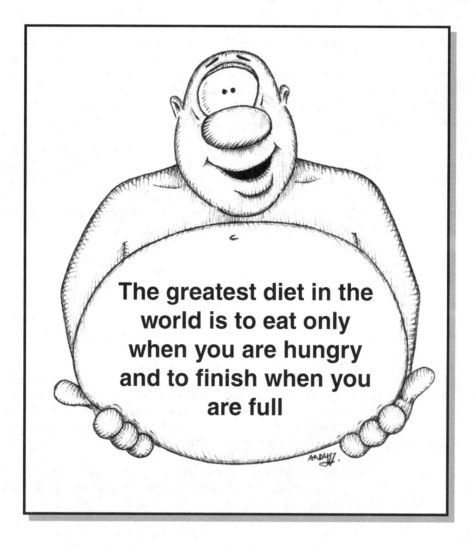

And I can tell you what the book isn't about. It isn't about pain and it isn't about calorie counting. The chances are you may have had enough of that already. Trust me, life's too short.

If you've never succeeded in losing weight before, it's just a question of finding the way that's right for you to do it. And there always is a way. Many people think that if they've tried to diet and failed, the problem lies with their own lack of will power or determination. There's a temptation to think that it must be just a question of applying the same old methods – harder, longer, or with more determination.

It's a temptation, certainly, but don't give in to it. The hard truth is that if you always do what you've always done, you'll always get what you've always got. It's like watching a fly, buzzing around inside a window. It will throw itself at the window time and time again until it falls, exhausted, to the window sill. A few feet away there's probably an open door. There's no point in throwing yourself again and again at the same bit of double glazing. If one way out didn't work for you before, don't risk disappointment, burnout or injury by making the same mistake again. Stop, review the situation and look for the open door.

The difference that will make the difference is what you do with the ideas I give you. Some will work for you better than others. Take the time you need to find out which of these exercises and suggestions will really help you change your life.

Chapter Two

Getting To Know You

It was a while before I talked to Lisa at the club again. I was busy with my new development, the Pete Cohen weight control programme and, to be honest, I was pretty nervous around Lisa since she had collapsed. I couldn't just take her for granted the way I'd done before. I didn't see her strong and slim the way I used to. She looked frail and thin to me, and seeing her working out at the club made me uncomfortable. She'd never looked as if she needed to diet anyway - Mo on the other hand ... but I figured Mo was happy the way she was.

When I'd originally suggested to Lisa that she might start exercising I really thought it might take her mind off dieting. It never occurred to me that she'd get obsessional about exercising as well as about eating.

"Obsessional." That was it! I was just about to lock up for the night but I went right back into the office on a surge of inspiration and set up the PC. It didn't take long and I was pretty pleased with the printout. I stuck it straight up on the board ready for the next morning.

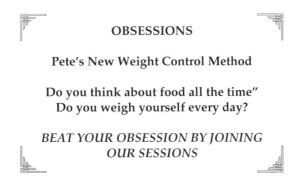

OBSESSIONS

Pete's New Weight Control Method

Do you think about food all the time"
Do you weigh yourself every day?

BEAT YOUR OBSESSION BY JOINING
OUR SESSIONS

Then I went home.

The next week I had a surprise. It was at the start of the first obsessions group. Fifteen people had turned up, and it was an interesting mix of die-hard dieters and newcomers to the wonderful world of weight control. Just as I was about to introduce myself and explain what we were going to cover in the first session, two men in track suits crashed in through the side door. For a minute I thought two of the bouncers from the bar in the next building had come through the wrong entrance, but then I recognised one of them. It was Ben.

He was out of breath. 'Hi, Pete,' he said, 'sorry we're late, why don't you just continue with everybody else and we'll weigh ourselves in here.'

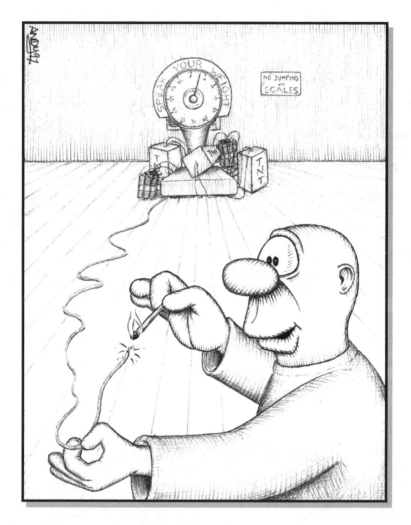

What Are You Weighting For?

'You don't have to weigh in,' I told them. 'I've done away with the weekly weigh so nobody has to rush to the loo at the last minute or drink coffee all afternoon. All the normal pre-slimming group activities are OUT. You come as you are and while you're in this room we are not going to talk about scales or dieting or any of that other negative stuff.' A Barbara Windsor look-alike (only the waistline was missing) in the front row put her hand up.

I nodded at her 'Yes, Faye?'

'If we don't weigh ourselves every week, how are we going to know whether we're losing weight or not? I'm hoping to get some new ideas because, frankly, none of the other groups have done much for me, but we've got to know how we're doing surely? It's not going to be very motivational otherwise, is it?'

The lady next to her chimed in. 'Faye's right. It's all about motivation. That's what was wrong with the last group. She didn't motivate us really, did she? But I thought the weighing in was really great. There was usually somebody worse than me so I didn't feel so bad.'

'Except the last three sessions when you put on two pounds every time,' said Faye. 'That's why you said we should leave. Right?'

I thought I could see what the other slimming group leader might be up against. Just getting these two to stop talking was going to be a challenge.

'I want to start by explaining to you that this group isn't about comparing yourself to anybody else. It's about getting to know yourselves better, getting to know when you're hungry, what you need to eat and how you need to exercise. It's about taking back responsibility for your own body and learning to feel good about yourself.'

'Sounds like a feminist self awareness group to me,' said Ben's friend. 'I admit I need to lose a few pounds, but I'm not convinced that this is the right place for me to do it. I'll be honest with you,' he added aggressively, 'I want a straightforward workout and a diet sheet, not a lot of airy-fairy mind games.'

I could see that some of the women were getting a bit annoyed with him so I went for the jugular: 'It's my guess that you're an ex-rugby player like Ben? Am I right?'

He nodded.

'I don't know what you do now,' I continued, 'but you know damn well that if you want a diet sheet and a work-out you can get that from your old training schedules, or you can just sign up at the gym and we'll put something together for you. I can't believe you haven't tried all the standard methods already, and you haven't stuck to any of them, have you?'

He sat down again, looking annoyed. 'OK, nothing's worked so far. Let's give you a try.'

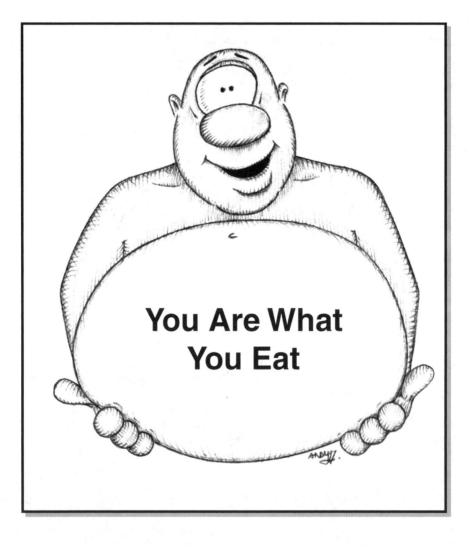

The rest of the session went quite well. I talked them through some basic information about dieting and why it doesn't work for 98% of the people who try it. Then I got them thinking about their own motivation and what they actually wanted for themselves at the end of the eight sessions. Before I knew it I was giving them their food diary for the first week and saying goodbye.

I was just taking the chairs out and setting up the room for the last aerobic session of the day when I noticed both Lisa and Mo at the back of the class. Actually, it was hard to miss them. Lisa was wearing an amazing lime green outfit. She looked like she ought to be up front, not lurking in the back row. I guessed she was there to support Mo who was wearing a shiny black track suit, although it could have been a couple of bin liners. The pair of them would have made perfect 'Before' and 'After' pictures in Slimmer of the Week.

For once, Lisa was smiling and Mo looked anxious. It was usually the other way round. 'Don't worry,' said Lisa. 'I'm not going to faint on you again. I had some lunch. Promise. What's more,' she added, 'you can stop avoiding me. What happened wasn't your fault. I've got it under control now.'

'Got what under control?'

'Me, I suppose.'

'I'll take your word for it' I turned to Mo. 'What the hell are you doing here? You usually ask me why I don't get a proper job instead of hanging around all day in black lycra while women admire my muscles.'

'We'll talk later,' said Lisa. 'See you in the Duke's Head when you've locked up.'

I went to the front and started the class. I was uneasy. I had a feeling I was about to find out some more about this diet problem that was going to make my neat and tidy solutions look less than perfect.

They got to the pub before me and I joined them in a corner of the bar. Mo looked exhausted. I guessed she'd pushed herself too hard trying to keep up with Lisa, but I didn't like to say anything.

Lisa made room for me 'Hi, Pete. Great exercise class, but you've got to get that bloody poster down.'

'What poster? You don't mean my weight control group? I only just put that one up, as a matter of fact, I think it's pretty clever.'

'Can't you see, it really annoys people like me?' said Lisa. 'You're implying that everyone who watches their weight is obsessional and dysfunctional.'

'You mean mad,' said Mo. She was being unusually quiet and I noticed she'd only ordered herself a half.

If you want to be
slimmer, fitter and
healthier, make the
decision to change

Get the right information

Commit to achieving
your goal

Then cut yourself off
from all other
possibilities

'I don't mean mad, of course I don't. I've just noticed that half the people who come to the club don't come because they want to be fit and healthy and feel good, they come because they think they've got to sweat and suffer to get thin. That's a high proportion of my membership and they don't seem to talk or think about anything else but food and weight. They talk to me about it all the time. I hear them talking to each other about it all the time. They count pounds, they count calories, they'd count units of pain if they could. But they don't get any thinner.'

'Well that's good for you then.' Mo was with us again. 'It means they keep coming and you make more money.'

'It's not good for me. Why do you think we have such a high drop out rate? Because exercise is too damned painful if you do it for the wrong reasons. You can't keep something up if you focus on the pain of it. I want people to lose the weight they want to lose and then keep coming because it's fun for them. I want them to feel good about themselves and get pleasure from the exercise ...'

'Yeah, yeah, we all know you have a dream. You make it sound like Disneyland Paris' said Lisa, 'but that's not the point I was making. Just because I weigh myself regularly and watch my diet, that doesn't make me obsessional. And, you've got to admit that I look OK on it.'

I've been around long enough to realise that when someone, male or female, says 'Do I look OK?' what they really mean is 'Do I look wonderful?', so I knew what to do with this one.

'You look terrific. You always do. But answer me this. Do you honestly feel as good as you look?'

'Below the belt' muttered Mo.

'Let's just drop it, alright?' Lisa was looking cornered 'I'll have another diet Coke if you're buying.'

'Are you having a pint, Mo?'

'No, get me the same as Lisa this time.'

When I got back with the drinks Mo had a question for me. 'What are you actually doing with all the fat ladies at your obsessional evenings? How about telling us the secret for free since we're your friends?'

'They're not all fat and they're not all ladies, and, before you ask, they're not all obsessional.'

'Alright, don't be so touchy, what do you actually do with them?'

The willingness to be slimmer comes from you

And you can do almost anything if you truly decide to

'Well, for a start, my aim is to get them to take decisions and run their lives for themselves rather than rely on a diet or an exercise plan, or even on me. So one of the first steps is to try and help people to understand themselves a bit better and like themselves a bit more. The first week I always ask them to start keeping a food diary.'

'Oh, wow!' said Lisa, 'big new breakthrough! I've lost count of how many diets I've been on where I had to write down everything I ate and count the calories and the grams of fat and...'

'No, that's not it. Listen, why don't you try it, just for a week, both of you. Humour me. Lisa, you're an expert on diets – you can be my focus group. Write down everything you eat, every biscuit, grape, crisp, Whopper, whatever, but it's just a list. You're not counting calories or anything else. It's like you were throwing everything you ate into a shopping trolley for a week to see what it looks like at the end.'

'Sounds better than throwing it all up down the loo,' said Lisa.

'Oh, God, you aren't doing that are you?'

'No, of course not, but there's a lot of it about. In fact it's almost respectable enough to be a recognised dietary technique. Hey, that's an idea, why don't you be the first person to write the Bulimia Diet Book?'

'That's not funny, it's sick!'

That broke the tension and we all fell about laughing. 'OK,' said Mo, when she'd recovered. 'What do we do with this backwards shopping list at the end of the week then?'

'I'll tell you when you've done it. Don't think about it, don't analyse it, just do it.'

I decided the atmosphere had relaxed enough for me to ask a few personal questions. 'What were you doing at the club, Mo? And what's all this about diet sodas and halves? You're acting really strange, and I don't know if I can cope with it!'

Lisa smiled. 'She's fallen in love.' She nudged Mo whose drink splashed on the bar.

'And what's that got to do with exercising?'

Mo looked really embarrassed. 'I just thought I'd have a go on Lisa's scales last week and I got a bit of a shock' she said. 'I'm two and a half stone more than last time I weighed myself.'

'When was that?'

'Oh, years ago, before I moved to London.'

'Can you believe that?' said Lisa. 'She hasn't weighed herself for three years. We worked it out! That is not normal.'

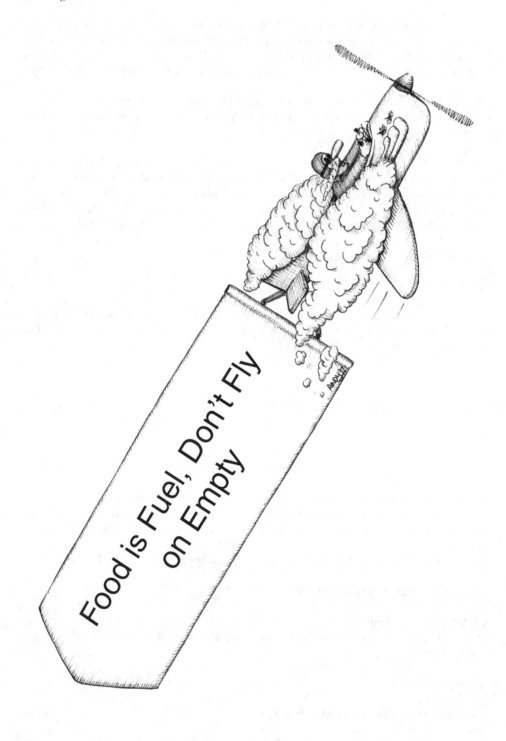

'Actually,' I said, 'it's fine. I think checking your weight every five minutes is pretty weird. I haven't even got any scales.'

'You're the odd one out then. Everyone has scales, and there's nothing wrong with just checking your weight twice a day,' said Lisa, 'It's like cleaning your teeth. Just tell me, what's the difference between doing that and looking in the mirror to check your lipstick's not smudged? How else would you know if you're on target?'

'If you can do up your jeans you're OK.'

'Oh no you're not,' said Mo. 'I've got an old pair of jeans I wear sometimes when I'm fixing the motorbike. I've had them for years.'

'Let's face it Mo, those jeans are hardly a fashion statement.'

The temperature was rising. I did my best. 'Mo, I've known you since we were at college. We've been drinking together, we've played tennis together, we've even been to the odd lecture. You honestly don't look any different to me now than you did then.'

Mo burst into tears. 'You mean I've always looked fat, even when I wasn't,' she sobbed.

I was beginning to feel like getting people wrong was becoming a habit. Lisa put an arm round Mo, and I tried to stop myself banging my head on the bar.

The barman leaned over. He was a regular at the club and I knew him pretty well. He nodded towards the girls 'Time of the month probably' he said.

A few days later, when I'd recovered, I took a really nice plant round to Mo and Lisa's flat. I wondered about a bottle of wine but decided I didn't want to know how many wasted calories there were in a bottle of Chardonnay and Lisa was bound to tell me.

I stood on the doorstep behind the pink geranium and inside I could hear raised voices. 'If it's him, tell him I'm not ready' that was Mo. Lisa's reply was unprintable but eventually she came to the door. She smiled at the plant and started to say 'Oh, how sweet' then she saw me. 'Oh, it's you' she said, and turned around. As she'd taken the plant and left the door open I reckoned it was the next best thing to being invited in, so I followed her.

When I got into the kitchen I realised they had a visitor.

I thought I'd better introduce myself. 'Hello, I'm Pete.' The visitor burst out laughing and turned around. It was Mo. Like I'd never seen her before.

Let me tell you about Mo. She's short and dark-haired and she bounces. She's definitely a pretty woman and she's definitely big, but I've never thought of her as fat because she's so lively.

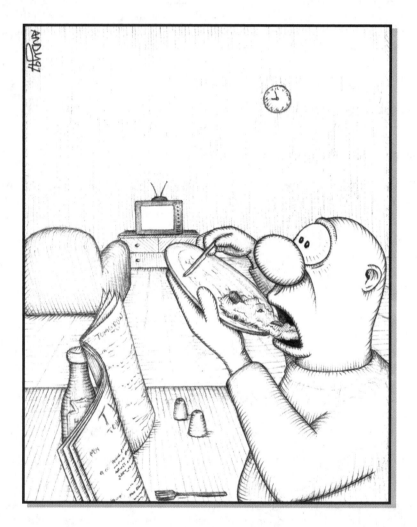

Calories Are Wasted If They Aren't Tasted

It was the first time I'd seen her wearing a dress, and make up, and nail varnish; she'd even let her hair down - literally. The effect was impressive. Lisa was laughing too. 'See,' she said, 'that's what a few weeks of weighing and calorie counting and exercising can do for a woman.'

Mo inspected the plant. 'And what's this chrysanthemum for?'

'Well, I sort of felt I ought to say sorry about Friday night. I still don't understand what happened so that probably makes it my fault. Anyway, I thought it was a geranium.'

'So,' said Lisa, 'you came round to apologise but you don't know what for. Maybe we need to talk after all. Sit down Mo, you can't get any readier than you are.'

Suddenly everything started clicking into place, about twenty hours late. 'Mo, you've got a new boyfriend. Who is it?'

'Nobody you know.'

'Well, you look beautiful but you always looked good anyway, and what's all this rubbish about getting fat. I see fat every day and, believe me, you're not.'

'I've put on two and a half stone. The scales don't lie. I know I put on some weight when I started up the catering business, but I kidded myself it was muscle and a lot of it is definitely fat.'

'It probably was muscle to start with,' I told her. 'You used to do a lot more of the cooking and delivery work yourself at the beginning didn't you? The last year or so I get the impression that you're supervising and marketing and going out to lunch with clients. Your lifestyle's changed, so it's hardly surprising that your weight's changing too.'

'I want to get rid of the fat and build the muscle,' said Mo. 'I'm not going for the heroin chic image. I'm going for the James Bond Woman look. I just don't want to turn into my mum twenty years too early.'

'Why are you trying to justify it to Pete?' Lisa was looking irritable. 'If you want to lose a couple of stone, just do it!'

'I'm not sure about a couple of stone,' I said. 'That seems a bit drastic, why not aim to trim off a stone and then see how you look and feel?'

Lisa intervened. 'It's no good setting your sights too low. I keep telling Mo it won't be easy. It never works if it's easy. She's got to aim high, otherwise she won't stick with it.'

They were both looking at me. I could see this visit going the same way as that session in the pub. I didn't know what to say. They knew I didn't know what to say. I felt like a Tom cat being watched by two tigers and I didn't want to make a sudden move.

DON'T THINK OF A PINK ELEPHANT

What happens if I tell you not to think of a pink elephant? Your brain has to produce one first and then delete it. If you say to yourself "I must not *keep eating*", or "I have to lose *this weight",* guess what message you get?

You will probably picture yourself carrying weight or eating food.

Your brain is like a heat seeking missile. It will go wherever you focus it.

How about telling yourself "I want to be *slimmer, fitter and healthier,"* or *"I want to feel more confident and have more energy."*

Tell yourself what you want, not what you don't want

Start putting your aims and goals and dreams for a slimmer future into positive terms. Imagine how an architect has to draw up detailed plans before starting to build a house. Your vision of how *you* want to be needs as much detail as the architect's drawings.

'How about a cup of tea?' I said. 'And don't offer me a biscuit unless it's got real chocolate on and I can have two of them. You can watch me eat them if you like.'

'There hasn't been a biscuit in this flat since Mo met *Him*' said Lisa. 'I've been missing them myself, I used to sneak a quick one when I got home from work sometimes.'

We both stared at her. 'You! Eating biscuits, you're kidding.'

'No, I'm not, I just used to miss dinner to make up for it.'

'You skipped dinner because of a couple of biscuits? That's crazy.'

'The truth will out. That's what you really think about me, isn't it? You think I'm mad and you think I'm a bad influence on Mo. You may as well admit it.'

'No, I don't. Of course I don't think anything like that. I just find it hard to believe that two intelligent, successful, beautiful women could be so negative.'

'What's negative about trying to stay slim? As far as I'm concerned, being negative means slobbing around in a track suit eating pizzas in front of the TV every night. I haven't quite got to that stage yet.'

We were all sitting down around the table now with our mugs of tea. I could tell that Mo was trying not to smudge her lipstick. I had their attention and I had one chance to keep it.

'If I say to you, "Don't think of a pink elephant", what happens?'

'Don't be silly, you know what happens.'

'OK, so what happens when you go to the bathroom and get on the scales?'

'I'm thinking about my weight, I'm wondering if I've gained a pound or two overnight – and believe me, that can happen!'

'Of course, but it's just fluid, so don't worry about it. Can't you see what you're doing? Every time you get on the scales, you're reinforcing that picture you have of yourself as a potential fat person. You're imagining yourself fat. You're focusing on FAT. I bet you have a fat picture of yourself, don't you? Haven't you ever heard of a self-fulfilling prophecy?'

'I don't see myself as being fat exactly,' said Mo, 'just dumpy, but lately I've been getting a lot more realistic feedback.'

Before I could ask her who she was getting the realistic feedback from, Lisa said, 'People are always telling me I'm slim and maybe I am. But what they don't know is that there is a fat version of me waiting to break out at any minute. Weighing myself is more than just checking, it's almost like a magic spell to ward off the evil. If I don't

MORE PINK ELEPHANTS

Thinking positively and striving towards clearly visualised goals doesn't come without practice. Most people find it much easier to formulate what they want to avoid. Like WEIGHT. Presumably that's why they join classes to watch it. It's not surprising the weight won't go away if you never let it out of your sight or get it off your mind.

Ask yourself:

What do I want?
What will that do for me?
How will I know that I've got what I want?

See how you would look, feel how you would feel if you were the way you want to be.

This, by the way, takes more practice for some people than for others

But with plenty of practice everybody can learn to do it

weigh myself, the pounds might creep on while I'm not looking. It's the same with the diet and exercising, I have to stick to some kind of ritual to prevent myself from suddenly turning into a blob of lard and dissolving on the carpet.'

'And don't look at me like that, Pete. You might think it's crazy, but I know plenty of people who are worse than me. In fact, it's official, I was reading in a diet book the other day about this experiment in America. They put 1000 women in a room that had three mirrors in it. Sounds bad, doesn't it? But it gets worse. One of the mirrors made them look slimmer.'

'Like the ones in dress shops,' said Mo.

'No, really, is that true? That's terrible.'

'I have a girlfriend who used to be a buyer for Selfridges. She never said they did it but apparently some of the big stores do.'

'Anyway' said Lisa, determined to finish her story, 'the second mirror made them look slightly larger and the third one was accurate. But 75% of the women believed the one that made them look fatter. So, you see' she finished triumphantly, 'it's not just me.'

I was thinking about the time these people must be spending worrying about their size and shape, weighing themselves, counting calories, going to classes, dropping out of health clubs.

'They could be playing cricket or going fishing.'

'What?' They were both looking at me as if I was mad too.

'Sorry, thinking aloud. Tell me Lisa, have you ever weighed more than you do now? Since you were sixteen anyway?'

She reached for her purse and pulled out a bunch of photos. I recognised her Mum and Dad, a couple of ex-boyfriends and even her baby nephew. But there was one I hadn't seen before. For a minute I thought she must have a sister I hadn't met; there was certainly a resemblance. But this girl, standing on a beach somewhere wearing a bright red swimsuit and a sunhat was a big girl. Not exactly fat, but certainly statuesque. Lisa had gone one better than most people; she had a real fat picture of herself. Or so she thought.

'That's you, isn't it? How long ago?'

'Three years. It was before I moved in with Mo.'

'I've never seen it before,' said Mo. 'I thought you'd always been kind of wispy, the way you are now. I wouldn't say you were fat in that photo anyway, impressive is what I'd call you, a bit like Pamela Anderson. I wish I was tall. You don't know how lucky you are.' She stopped for breath. 'Why are you carrying a photo of yourself around anyway?'

The key to changing your eating habits is awareness

Look for the times that you eat during the day

How much are you eating?

Do you enjoy every bite?

What are your food choices?

'When I go to a restaurant or if I'm tempted to have a fat lunch at work, I nip off to the loo and have a look at it. I suppose it scares me into sticking to my diet.'

'That photo scares you???' both Mo and I were amazed.

The doorbell rang. This time, Mo didn't hesitate. She grabbed her bag and jacket and was gone.

Lisa and I looked at each other. 'Have you met him yet?' I asked her.

'No, she thinks I'd eat him' she paused 'And why not. After all, I eat just about anything, given half a chance.'

'As we're on the subject of food, did you and Mo do anything about that food diary I asked you to try out?'

Lisa looked a bit sheepish. 'I don't know about Mo, but I thought you had a point when you asked me to give it a try. After all, I have to be one of the world's greatest experts on diets that don't work so I thought I would give you the benefit of my opinion. After all, you must be so busy telling other people what to do that you probably don't have much time to read up on what the competition is doing.'

'Wrong, Lisa. I'm willing to bet that I've read more diet books than you have – after all, I only read them, it's bound to take you longer if you're trying them all out.'

I was pleased to see that Lisa looked impressed. 'I'm impressed,' she said 'And what do you think of them?'

'I think the big problem with most of them is that they stick to formulas and ignore people. A lot of them are common sense but they don't tell people how to personalise the methods and a few of them are actually dangerous. Fortunately, the really wacky ones tend to be so difficult to follow that there isn't much chance of anyone following them to the letter and doing themselves any harm.'

'That's depressing, but why don't they work?'

'Because they don't take account of pleasure and pain and they can't know what motivates each individual reader. Take this food diary for example. All I'm trying to get you to do with that is learn more about yourself, why you eat, when you eat and what exercise means to you. Now, come on, tell me how you got on with it?'

'Well, I wouldn't say this in front of Mo, but I had a few surprises. You know that thing about the biscuits? I discovered that the first thing I do when I come through the door at night is reach for the biscuit tin. In fact, I'm even thinking about that biscuit before I get off the train. It's like Pavlov's bloody dogs, I'm virtually salivating as I go down the steps looking for my keys. I've tried not having any in the house, but the corner shop by the station is always open and I go in for a paper and then it's just so easy to buy something to eat as well. In fact, if I don't ask for a Kit Kat, Mrs Patel usually hands one over anyway. She knows me that well!'

Did you know that 90% of people who buy a book don't read past the first chapter?

Well, talk about food for thought. As I walked down the street following our conversation, I was trying to reconcile all the contradictions. I still don't understand why sensible, successful people often don't see themselves the way other people see them. The daily double weigh-in and the low self-image problem weren't new to me. A lot of the men and women who came to my weight control groups were saying exactly the same things but most of them really were more than a few pounds overweight.

After a while I decided that I was asking myself the wrong question. After all, 'Why' is none of my business. How, and what and where and when, that's much more to the point. One thing I have learned is that 'why' questions hardly ever get useful answers.

So, what were Lisa and Mo doing that was making weight control such a chore? If you can answer these questions at the beginning of the war against weight, you've definitely won the first battle. By the way, you have probably already realised by now that my approach is as much to do with how you think about yourself as it is about what you do.

That's why the thing about the scales is important. Lisa admitted that every time she got on the scales the uppermost thought in her mind was weight. So she's spending a lot of energy focusing on the very thing she wants to get rid of. That's the trouble with scales; they focus you on the wrong thing. They aren't good for positive thinking.

Another problem with scales is that they don't discriminate. They can't tell if they're registering an increase in fat, fluid or muscle. They don't know what time of the month it is (if you're a woman). They don't know about your muscle mass and tone or your weight distribution. They certainly don't know if you're on a diet – and scales are almost guaranteed to slow down your metabolism. My advice is to trust the scales less and trust yourself more. If you really can't bear to throw them out, try not to use them more than once every six or eight weeks. Some people say it's harder than giving up smoking and I believe them. I think there ought to be a government health warning printed on bathroom scales.

After all, there are lots of other ways to measure your success. You can start to look and feel better, like Mo did, even before the weight starts to fall away. You can learn to listen to your body telling you when and what to eat, you will know when you can run up the escalator without feeling breathless and you'll certainly know when you aren't afraid to look in the mirror any more.

Before we move on to the exercises for this session, I should just tell you that the first thing I did when I went into the club next day was to tear down the notice that had offended Mo and Lisa. "Lighten Up with Pete" read the new one. Obsessions were out and Positive Thinking was in.

Chapter Three

What You Really Want

I saw Mo again a few days later at the club. She looked more like her old self but I noticed she was wearing more make-up and the heels were getting higher. 'You'll be taller than me soon,' I said. 'How's the new man?'

She changed the subject immediately. 'Lisa and I want to sign up for your Lighten Up programme or whatever you call it. We'll be bringing a friend along. When's the next session?'

'Well, you've missed the first session, but we've been talking about some of the stuff I do in that so you should catch up. Next Friday at 7.30, alright? And who's your friend? Someone I know?'

'Don't be so nosy. Just put down three places, OK?'

'Hang on, before you go, just tell me why the sudden interest in my classes? I've been getting a hard time from you two about my weight control programme.'

'Lisa and I have decided you might have a few good ideas. That pink elephant thing for example. Do you run some exercises about that positive thinking stuff?'

'Of course I do, this class isn't just about dieting and exercising you know, there are all kinds of hippie mind control exercises involved as well. In fact, if you asked me what was the single most important factor in my weight loss system, it would be the pink elephant.'

'What, more important than what you eat and how much you sweat?'

'Yes, because your body will follow what your mind tells it to do. If you spend time programming your body but you haven't bothered to get your head round it first, of course you're going to fail. That's why so many diets don't work, because people haven't checked it out with themselves first. You always get what you focus on, so if you focus constantly on fat and calories, that's what you'll get. You'll get fatter, ultimately, because you won't be able to stop yourself thinking about all those wonderful, forbidden calories. Remember Descartes?'

'You mean what he really said was, "I think fat, therefore I am fat"?' Mo dug me in the ribs, 'you've sold me the pink elephant. And, by the way, I don't know about Lisa, but I did start keeping a Food Diary. I had to give it up though.'

'Why?'

'Much too scary. It told me all sorts of things I didn't really want to know.'

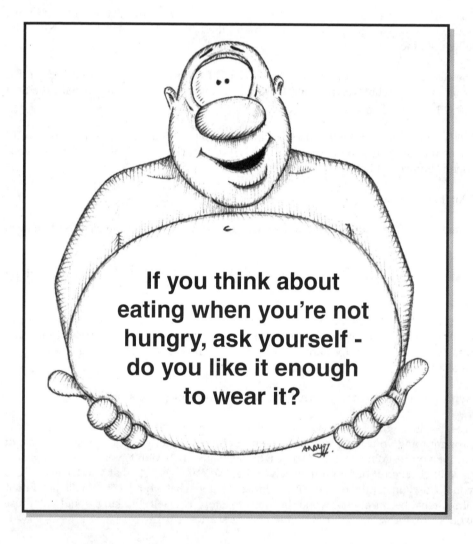

'If it told you anything you didn't know already, that's one of the things it's meant to do.'

'Yes, but I don't see the point of just counting up how many digestives with peanut butter I can get through in a day. Just knowing it makes me feel worse, not better.'

'Surely it's better that you're the first to know if you're eating too many of them. Let's face it, the rest of the world is going to find out sooner or later.'

'How come? Your big selling pitch on this diary was that it's confidential.'

'Yes, but if you really are eating too much peanut butter or whatever, sooner or later you're going to be wearing it, aren't you?'

Mo glanced down at her hips which were cleverly disguised by an expensive-looking loose tunic over a long skirt with a matching scarf. 'I'm wearing it already,' she said, sadly. 'And carrying it up and down stairs, it's almost as bad as being pregnant and trying to hide it. In fact, if I was pregnant it would be a lot easier because I'd get sympathy and time off work and a seat on the tube.'

'And ultimately a lot of sleepless nights. Mo, I'm not trying to depress you. It looks to me like you've lost quite a few pounds already, and you haven't been working on it for long, have you? I'm more worried about you trying to lose too much too fast. You can't just stop eating and start exercising overnight. Your body will try and save you from starvation by slowing down your normal fat-burning rate.'

'Oh great, that's all I need. My own metabolism's programmed to sabotage me!' She stepped towards me and put her hand on my shoulder. 'Pete, I know what you're saying, and I really appreciate your concern. But I'm really trying to be sensible about it. Just stop worrying. I only started a few weeks ago after the big weigh in we told you about. And I haven't lost much yet, it's more a question of re-packaging if you know what I mean.'

'Well the re-packaging's impressive. Are you sure you really need to lose two and a half stone?'

'Nope. I'm going for three. You know the other night, at the aerobic class? Well, from my viewpoint at the back, I could see all these perfect bums and thighs in front of me zapping around to the music and I couldn't even keep up. That was bad enough. Then, when I got back to the changing room and caught sight of myself in the mirror I thought it was Michelin Woman. I'm getting rid of that track suit, but not till I've lost the first two stone.'

'You certainly didn't look too good in the pub afterwards' I said. 'And I'm not surprised. You hadn't done anything like that for a while, had you? You didn't have to try and keep up with all those people who are doing it several times a week. Lots of people stop exercising before they've even got started. Believe me, I know, I see it every week. They try it once or twice and it's so painful they give up for ever. But exercise doesn't have to be painful. If it hurts you'll be more tired than exhilarated afterwards and you might be burning more sugar than fat. You've just got to respect

DAYDREAM PRACTICE

Imagination is more important than knowledge

Albert Einstein

Everybody daydreams. Some people are better at it than others but, whether it comes naturally or not, you can become a wide-screen, Technicolor expert if you concentrate.

Yes, I'm actually saying you need to work harder at your daydreaming technique. Visualise the person you want to be. It's a movie with you as the Director and Star.

There is a theory that to fix something in your mind, you need to repeat it at least twenty times.

You could see how well this works for you.

your body a bit more. Start slowly, work up to the right pace for you gradually. You'll start feeling great, it's exhilarating, when you do it right. Like those Nike adverts. And, best of all, your body goes on burning off the fat long after you've stopped doing the leg lifts.'

'Well, for a start that sounds like crap to me. Lisa's been going to exercise classes since we started flat sharing and I haven't noticed her come bouncing back afterwards full of energy. She usually crawls into the kitchen and raids the bread bin. Two cheese sandwiches later and already she's miserable for the rest of the night. I've told her, she could save money by giving the class and the sandwiches a miss because as far as I can tell, the one cancels out the other.'

'She's overdoing it. We talked about that, remember? When she collapsed at the club? I'm trying to tell you it shouldn't be like that. Exercise and a good diet doesn't have to mean misery and deprivation. That's what I've been trying to get across to Lisa as well.'

'I'm not going to get like Lisa, I've got it all under control.' She walked off. Slower than usual and with her head down.

I didn't try and call her back. It was Wednesday and I usually go round to Ben's flat to watch the mid-week game. This Wednesday I'd had a better offer so I stopped by on my way to the wine bar to let him know I wouldn't be staying. I carried my bike down the basement steps and leaned it against the dustbins. The back door was open as usual and I could hear voices. I tried to push open the living room door but something was blocking it. Somebody yelled 'Is that the pizza?'

'No,' I shouted back, 'it's me.' I shoved the door hard enough to shift the cans that seemed to have stacked up behind it. 'Why don't you just phone the council and suggest they move the recycling bank round here?'

Five men were stretched out in front of the TV. Ben's friend was there, the one he'd brought to the aerobics class.

'Pete! Where have you been?' Ben looked up but didn't get up, 'you're late. Lucky the pizza is too. We ordered you some.'

'I'm not staying, I'm meeting somebody at Oscar's.'

There was a chorus of catcalls. I tried to change the subject. 'I don't see much point in aerobics and special diets if you are going to carry on like this every time there's some football on. You can't tell me that pizza and, what's this?' (I picked a large, empty bag off the floor,) 'cheese nachos, are allowed on the food combining diet, are they?'

Ben's friend from the aerobics class stood up and came over to me 'I ought to introduce myself,' he said, 'since Benjamin's not going to. I'm Lewis — and I've put a stop to all this bloody diet nonsense. Not eating chips with your steak is one of the stupidest ideas he's ever come up with and he used to be well known for stupid ideas when we were students. I've told him, I'm not eating out with him again if he's going to carry on like that.'

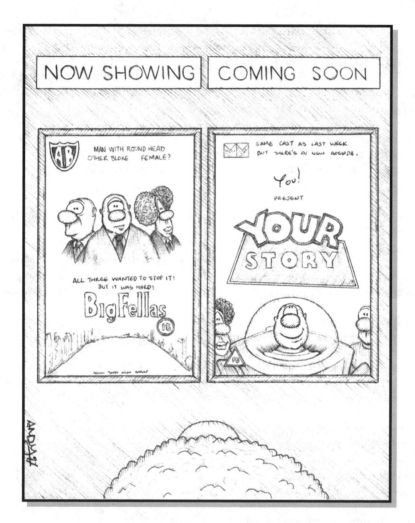

Daydreaming With Intent

Ben laughed. 'Lewis and I used to play for the same team, but we lost touch. I didn't see him for ages, then we end up sitting next to each other at the rugby club annual dinner. I haven't had such a good time for so long. Honestly Pete, you have no idea how much I had missed real food. I have come to the conclusion that life is just too short.'

'But I could see why he was doing it,' added Lewis. 'I didn't recognise him at first. I thought "who's that fat git up at the bar, he looks familiar?" and it was Ben! I couldn't believe it. I told him, 'It's nothing to do with your diet, mate, it's just lack of exercise. It's my mission to get you back into shape.' Then I found out it was worse than I'd thought ...'

Lewis was warming up to his subject and he had everybody's attention. I suspected he liked an audience and I could tell he didn't like me. I decided to let him have centre stage for a few more minutes until I judged the time was right to pitch in and give him the benefit of my opinion on a subject I knew a lot more about than him.

He continued, 'Yes, a lot worse than I thought. We had quite a few beers at the club dinner, and he can't take it like he used to. He told me everything.' He paused.

Everybody was leaning forward now, beer cans in hand, the television forgotten.

'I found out,' announced Lewis dramatically, 'that he's been sneaking off to weight control classes with a bunch of bloody women in St Mark's Hall.'

Everybody laughed. Ben looked miserable. 'I'd already decided to give up that food combining diet,' he said, 'and I admit this weight loss group was not my scene at all. We all had to weigh ourselves in front of everybody else and admit what we'd eaten that we shouldn't have. It was more like true confessions than weight control – the kind of thing my Auntie would go to. Anyway, I saw your notice Pete, and I said to myself that any class you ran had to be better than spending Friday evenings being ordered about by Mrs Hitler. So, I said to Lewis, "Before you start sneering at it, give it a try. It's all very well being rude about my beer gut, but you're not as thin as you used to be either".'

'I'm a prop forward, I'm not meant to look like a bloody fairy,' protested Lewis.

'You are not a prop forward, Man. You're a software engineer. You haven't played anything more energetic than snooker for the last two years. Stop kidding yourself.'

This was getting really interesting. I took a closer look at Lewis. He was certainly big, six foot five at least I would have thought, but he wasn't all muscle. He was wearing a fashionably baggy suit that made him look pretty impressive. I privately thought he was probably about twenty stone when he should have been around fourteen. Still, it was none of my business, or was it?

'So what did you think of my group?' I asked him. 'You rushed off so fast afterwards I didn't get a chance to talk to you.'

JUMP START YOUR SYSTEM

Start eating more fresh foods

Your body knows what to do with them and copes with them much more readily than with chemically altered, food-like alternatives

He looked at me for the first time. He hadn't said much at the group. 'I hear you're a fitness expert when you're not being a fatness expert,' he said.

I sensed a male challenge situation building up. I suspected Lewis had his own agenda and I wasn't very interested in it. But I wasn't about to let him get away with a remark like that. 'That's right,' I said. 'Why don't you come and work out at the club some time? I think we could set up a programme for you that will have you back in shape in, well, in your case, maybe six months.'

I didn't wait for a reply. I called over my shoulder, 'Got to go,' and went out to get my bike.

The following day I was in the office printing out schedules, when I suddenly noticed that the room I used on Friday nights for the slimming group and the aerobics was already booked. 'Hang on.' I said to Jane, who was eating her sandwiches while she caught up with some paperwork, 'You can't do that, I always have the River Room on Fridays.'

'It's not me,' she said. 'I don't even work Friday evenings, let me have a look at that.'

I passed the list across to her. 'That onion's a bit strong, I hope you haven't got any one-to-one clients this afternoon.'

She stopped chewing and sniffed. 'I suppose it is a bit, I hadn't noticed. I'm trying to get this membership list sorted out. You've put me right off it now!'

'You mean you didn't even know what you were eating.'

'Oh, come on Pete, you know what it's like, I've had a hectic morning, I've got two classes this afternoon, I need to eat.'

'Sure, but it seems a shame not to enjoy it.'

She gave me a V sign and looked at the paper I'd given her. 'I can tell you who that is. You know that woman who used to run slimming classes at the church hall? Well, apparently it's been closed down for re-wiring. They don't want to risk electrocuting the brownies. So she's renting space from us.'

'How could you do that! You knew damn well I was starting our own slimming groups right here, in the same room, on the same night! What is going on here!'

'Don't blame me,' she passed back the booking list. 'I didn't take the booking. Anyway, you know we're supposed to try and rent out as much space as we can. There are the two rooms on the second floor, what's wrong with one of them? It's not as though you need any special equipment and I'm sure the calorie counters won't care.'

'Well I care. That top floor's bloody depressing, it needs decorating.'

'Exactly,' said Jane, 'we can't really rent it out at the full rate till we do.'

Rather than measuring your success by how much you weigh, ask yourself:

Do I feel better?

Do I feel slimmer?

How are my clothes fitting me?

Do I have more energy?

Am I eating when I'm hungry?

'But I can use it, because my groups don't matter I suppose. And what happens if they end up in the wrong room?'

'You mean they might prefer it – is that what's worrying you? We've already had one phone call from a customer who said she didn't think much of your slimming class because she didn't get weighed. She thought you weren't taking her seriously.'

I thought I knew who it was. Faye at a guess. I made a mental note to call her later. Meanwhile, I had to let everybody know the venue had changed and get some notices up for the evening. I was about to leave when I remembered Faye again and rang her. She was embarrassed, So was I. But, as I said, 'If you're not happy with the way I'm doing things, I'd rather talk it over with you now than try and discuss it in front of everybody else at the next group.'

'Oh Pete, I'm sorry, I didn't actually phone up to complain you know. I just called your office because I thought you said we were starting early next week and I wanted to check the time. Then, when I got through, that young lady asked me if the classes were working for me. Well, when she put it like that, I had to say no because, to be honest with you, the scales are showing up an extra couple of pounds since we started.'

'I thought I told you all, no weighing for a few weeks,' I reminded her. 'Scales are dangerous. They can ruin your whole day.'

'I didn't mean to, it was just that I was actually starting to feel better, you know, less breathless on the stairs, I could do up the top button on my uniform skirt, that sort of thing, so I thought I'd treat myself to a little weight check on Sunday night and I pulled the scales out from the cupboard again. I'd even put them away! Honestly! So I was really disappointed to see I'd gained when I thought I was losing. You've got to admit, it's disheartening.'

'That's exactly why I tell you to stay away from the scales, Faye. For one thing, fluid retention makes frequent weighing totally unreliable and, for another thing, you have to start building up muscle in order to burn off more fat. And muscle weighs a lot more. Sod the scales. Trust your feelings, trust your waistband, trust yourself a bit more. Your body knows what your ideal weight is.' I couldn't tell whether she was crying or laughing but I made her promise to come to the next group before I rang off.

So it was quite a bit later, following a busy afternoon, that I found myself cycling past Mo and Lisa's flat on the way home. Almost without thinking I got off the bike and chained it up to their gate.

Lisa let me in. 'Come on in.' She dashed back down the stairs. Mo was curled up on the sofa 'Hi,' she said without looking up. 'Have a seat and shut up. It's EastEnders time.' She passed me her bag of crisps and Lisa pushed the salsa dip in front of me.

As the credits came up on the screen the crisp packet came past me again. 'No thanks, they taste like cardboard. What are they?'

'Low fat crisps,' said Lisa. 'They're good for you.'

WORKING FROM YOUR OWN BLUEPRINT

If we are overweight it may be because we've interfered with our natural body design by eating too much and exercising too little...

How do you know what your natural blueprint is? Most people have lost track of it for so long, they've no idea where to find it or how to read it. Some people actually work very hard at re-wiring their personal circuits. Permanent dieters and exercise addicts and people with anorexia and bulimia spend hours of effort and concentration every day in an exhausting battle with themselves.

Fortunately, it's very hard to completely erase your personal plan. As long as you're still breathing, the blueprint, however faint, will be there.

Of course, that's why diets don't work...

Mo shook her head. 'No they're not, they're just not quite as bad for you as normal crisps. The trouble is, Pete's right, they do taste like cardboard, that's why you need to dip them in something otherwise they wouldn't be worth eating.'

'Why bother at all?' I asked her.

'I had a long, hard day – I need to relax and eat something in front of the TV. It takes my mind off everything.'

Lisa must have seen the look that crossed my face. She jumped up and hugged me. 'You're so transparent Pete. Wait for it Mo. Stand by your Food Diary! It's inspection time.'

'No it's not,' I felt annoyed. 'Just because I said those crisps weren't worth eating doesn't mean I'm criticising you. I need to get home and have dinner. I just called in to let you know about the change of venue for the slimming group.'

'Hey, don't give us a hard time. While you're here, lets just talk about it for a minute.' Lisa rushed out of the room and came back with a notebook which she opened. 'I've really got into this food diary now. And, guess what, I've started to see patterns — you know, like the Kit Kat after work that I told you about?'

'How many times have I told you, you've got a naturally obsessional personality,' Mo muttered, almost to herself.

Lisa didn't notice. 'The thing that bothers me about it is that, sure, it's interesting, but where is it going? I mean, usually you have to calculate calories and work out how many you're having per day. This diet is like working in the dark. No scales, no calories, it's like ten pin bowling when you can't see the pins.'

'It's not a diet,' I said. 'It's about getting back to your own natural blueprint. You know how you're doing when your body digests what you eat quickly and tells you when it's had enough. Oh, and when you start to be more active without having to make a big effort over it.'

They were both staring at me blankly so I continued: 'Calorie counting is a red herring. A calorie isn't a magic formula. It's just a unit of heat. That's how they were originally measured, by burning them, literally. It doesn't matter how many you take in, it's how many you burn. So, since nobody can burn an infinite number of calories, you might as well get the ones you need from food that's a) good for you and b) you enjoy.'

Mo shook her head. 'That is a contradiction in terms! Food you enjoy is never good for you. It's the sort of thing your mother tells "it's nothing that a bowl of chicken soup won't cure", but I'm old enough to know better than that now.'

LISTEN TO YOUR STOMACH

Our stomachs contain sensory nerves that can communicate very effectively with our brains, if they're given a chance. They tell us when we're hungry and thirsty and when we're satisfied.

Overweight people have learned how to override this system and replace it with a bunch of (usually bad) habits.

In order to lose weight we need to look out for these signals and listen to our stomachs so that we can start co-operating with our own bodies again. Eating's important enough to give it your full attention. After all, you wouldn't watch television while you were making love – would you?

'Well, I don't know about the chicken soup, but the idea that only things you hate are good for you is complete rubbish. It's like the old myth about 'no pain no gain' – actually I suppose it ought to be 'no pain no loss' but it doesn't rhyme. Take that bag of crisps for example. Just tell me, what was the point in them? You didn't really enjoy them - at least not without a load of salsa on them. I bet you didn't even taste half of them.'

'That's true,' said Lisa. 'Once she's watching something she's really addicted to, I could swap her crisps for a bag of the cat's treats and she wouldn't notice.'

Mo looked up. 'You haven't, have you?'

Lisa paused for a moment, watching the expression on Mo's face. 'No, I haven't, but it's crossed my mind. They're probably quite nutritious. Added vitamins and so on. I suppose they might be made out of fish flavoured mad cows though — that would be a bit of a drawback. And the cat probably wouldn't fancy those Lite Cocktail Snax.'

'Here's a revolutionary idea for you,' I said, 'why not try eating when you're hungry?'

'What does hungry feel like?' asked Mo.

'I can remember feeling hungry, when I used to go to dancing classes after school,' said Lisa. 'I didn't have time to go home for tea first so we used to buy chips and eat them at the bus stop afterwards. We used to just sit in the bus shelter and eat them and nobody said anything until we'd finished. They tasted absolutely wonderful, nothing tastes that good any more.'

'I tell you what,' I suggested. 'how about just stopping for a minute, before you eat something, anything, even a biscuit, and asking yourself how hungry you are on a scale of one to ten. One would be 'not at all hungry' and ten would be 'absolutely ravenous'.'

Lisa looked at me with blonde disdain. She was good at that. 'If we don't even know if we're hungry any more, how the hell are we going to know how hungry we are?'

Mo smiled suddenly. 'There are some feelings I could definitely give you a rating on,' she said.

Lisa put her hand over Mo's mouth and looked up at me over her shoulder. 'Well, Pete, or should I call you 'Source of all Dietary Wisdom'? How do you do that?'

'Mo's got a point. Take a feeling, any feeling. It doesn't have to be hunger, and I don't want to know what it is. At least, I do, but we'll get side-tracked. Just get a feeling in your minds, right? Imagine yourself in a situation where there's something you want to do. Have a hot bath, take a nap, get some fresh air, listen to music, anything. Could you put a rating on how much?'

'Yes, yes, yes,' yelled Mo.

THE HUNGER SCALE

1	2	3	4	5	6	7	8	9	10
Not		Fairly		Hungry		Very Hungry		Starving	

Every time you eat, ask yourself how hungry you are. If you score 5 or below, the chances are that you aren't really hungry at all.

Do something else instead of eating

Lisa had was shaking her head and looking dubious. 'Pay the phone bill, rating zero. Is that the kind of thing you mean?'

'You've got a right to be sceptical. Just give it a try for a week. Then give me a verdict. Meanwhile, how about buying a really nice bag of something absolutely delicious – like those cheese flavoured kettle chips for example — and just having a few of them, on their own, when you're not doing anything else. Don't you ever concentrate on what you're eating and really enjoy it?'

'I don't,' admitted Lisa. 'When I'm eating something healthy, I just eat it because I have to and I hope it's going to fill me up and stop me eating anything that's not so good for me. Then, when I eat something I really like, a Dime bar for example, I stuff it down as fast as I can in case I feel guilty in the middle of it and stop myself. Mind you, it's not so easy now I'm writing it all down. Sometimes I look at the list for the day and I think 'Oh my God, how did I eat all that?' and I end up going for another jog before bedtime.'

'Oh, that explains it,' said Mo. 'I wondered where you were the other night when I came in late. I looked round your door and your bed was empty but in the morning I heard you get up before me as usual.'

'I've got an idea for you,' I suggested, 'more of a challenge really. Why don't you both pick one of your eating patterns and see if you can change it before you start the group with me the week after next? OK Mo, I know you've given up on the diary, but just suppose you hadn't, what eating patterns would you be noticing? You could start with the EastEnders and crisps combination. Try watching it without the snacks.'

'What am I going to do with my hands?' asked Mo.

'Sit on them,' I said.

'Knit yourself one of those see-through tops and impress What's-His-Name,' suggested Lisa.

'And another thing,' said Mo, ignoring us. 'What about that blueprint theory? Look at me!' she threw up her arms, 'this is my blueprint. My Mum is this shape, my brothers are this shape and so is my cousin! Quite honestly, I'm not wild about this blueprint idea.'

'Alright, I admit, everybody is genetically different. Some families are more disposed to store fat than others. But, when it comes to the crunch, fat families don't just share DNA, they usually share lifestyles and eating habits too. You can still make a huge difference to your size and shape by adjusting what you eat and how much you exercise. Like I said, a calorie is just a measurement of heat. Some foods – like fat for example – have more calories.'

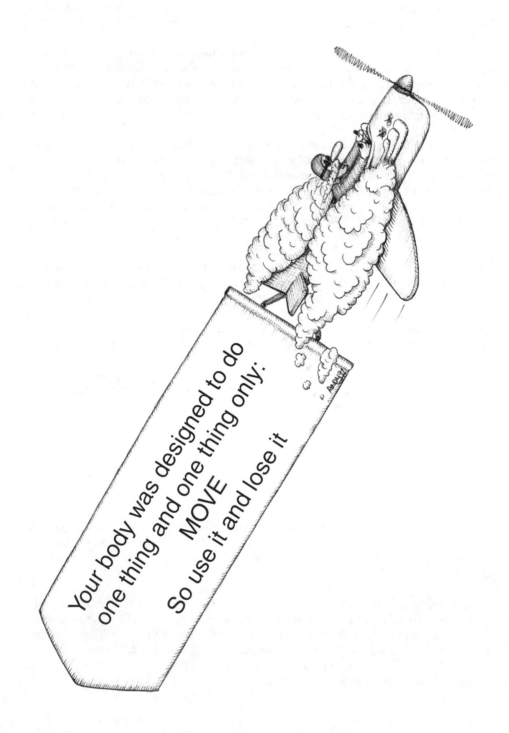

Your body was designed to do one thing and one thing only:
MOVE
So use it and lose it

'Exercise changes your body chemistry so that it doesn't have such a tendency to make fat out of the food you eat. And it sends out nutrients all around the body which then doesn't feel hungry because it's being supplied with energy. Fat, inactive people tend just to turn most excess nutrients into fat very quickly so they often feel hungry. You don't have to starve, just eat less fatty foods so you take in less calories and exercise more often so that you burn more as well.'

'Easy!' said Lisa. 'except that it isn't. I'm a weight loss veteran remember, I know you have to weigh and measure everything.'

'That isn't true Lisa. Just note down everything you eat, you'll soon have a pretty good idea of whether you're eating too much. The most important thing to be aware of is not the precise quantities but what sort of food you eat and whether you exercise regularly. The intake/exercise ratio is pretty crucial.'

'You've both admitted that a lot of the calories you take on board don't even get tasted, let alone enjoyed. Why not cut them out for a start? Don't eat unless you're over six or seven on the hunger scale. Just try making a few changes and log them in the food diary for a week. See what happens. Remember, calories tasted, not wasted.' I finished, smugly.

'You sound like the fascist cow who runs the slimming group at St Marks. Miriam. She's got lots of slogans like that. We're supposed to memorise them. I don't go to her any more because I thought spending three quid a week to be insulted wasn't a good use of my resources. I decided I could give myself a hard time at home, without any help from her.'

'Irritating woman,' said Mo. 'We did the catering for her daughter's wedding. She didn't just want sample menus, she wanted to know all the ingredients as well. It was a nightmare. She complained afterwards because she swore we'd put butter instead of low fat spread on the potatoes. Most people complain if they think we haven't. You'd think she'd have something else on her mind at her daughter's wedding. And you know the really funny bit? The daughter must be thirteen stone at least. The ultimate wedding meringue. Not much point in worrying about her figure at the reception. I said to Miriam, "you should have told her not to put butter on her potatoes six months ago, it's a bit late now," That didn't go down very well, but I'm not expecting repeat business so who cares.'

'Anyway,' said Lisa 'to get back to your helpful suggestion Pete, we'll have a go. But we're going to give you such a hard time if we don't look like Kate Moss at the end of the course.'

'Neither of you were ever meant to look like Kate Moss. I'm not convinced that Kate Moss is meant to look like Kate Moss but I'll reserve judgement on that since I don't know what she eats or what her family looks like. Remember the blueprint? Suppose I were to ask you to make a picture of yourself, not some supermodel, in your mind right now and describe it to me?'

SLIM PEOPLE

There are some things that slim people almost always do:

- Eat when they're hungry

- Stop eating when they're satisfied

- Notice how their bodies feel after eating.

Lisa looked up and into the distance. 'I can see myself, on a beach, I'm wearing a bikini and I'm running along the edge of the sea. I look really healthy, I'm laughing. God, it's like Baywatch.' Suddenly, she grabbed a cushion and stuck her head under it. 'Oh no, I don't believe it, it's me in that photo. That is NOT what I want.'

'That photo you carry around you mean? I think you look great in it. Maybe it is what you want.'

'No, it bloody well isn't. I'm huge in it. I'm just not good at creating images, that's all. I've got no imagination. I can't picture something unless I've actually seen it.'

'You surprise me,' said Mo. 'You have some pretty graphic dreams. I know, I have to listen to them at breakfast time. If they're for real you must have a secret life and I'd like to be in on it.'

When I left they were both in the kitchen preparing a mountain of salad. My suggestion that they might add some bread or rice, or even, shock, horror!, some chicken to it were ignored. I wondered how long it would take before the munchies struck after dinner. The trouble with living in town is that Seven Eleven is never far enough away and some of them are open twenty four hours now.

As I was going up the stairs to the door I called back to them both, 'Think of all that spare time you'll have left over when you stop eating, thinking about eating, counting calories and going to slimming classes! You could do something really exciting!'

I could just hear Mo shout after me 'Are you implying we're boring? I'll get you for that.'

As I cycled home I thought about Mo. She hadn't mentioned the new boyfriend and I guessed she wasn't planning to see him tonight. The lack of makeup, the old jeans and baggy T-shirt were all clues. It was funny how much difference she could make to herself without actually changing shape at all. I wondered whether it was really just packaging or whether her state of mind had a lot to do with how she looked as well.

I speeded up a bit. My stomach was telling me I needed to eat and that's a signal I don't like to ignore. I couldn't imagine what it would feel like not to know whether I was hungry or not. It must be terrible. It must be like not having control over your own life — or your own body. A bit like my ancient boiler in the flat. The thermostat went last winter and when I have the heating on the temperature is totally random, well, more like the palm house at Kew. So, of course, it's easier to turn it off than go to the trouble of getting it fixed. Maybe that's why nobody visits me after October. I made a resolution to call the heating engineer before next autumn came around. Some of my clients assume they can just pay me to fix their personal thermostats and speed up their metabolism for them. Unfortunately, everybody has to adjust their own. It's easy to do, but it takes some people a while to find it.

Chapter Four

Fat Burning Pills

The next day, of course, was Friday. The night of the Slimming Groups. Mine and Miriam's. I thought I'd better meet the lady I'd heard so much about so I looked into the River Room about twenty minutes before we were both due to kick off. I was expecting Margaret Thatcher in stretch jeans (Lisa had explained to me that slimming group leaders are supposed to be role models for their clients). The woman I saw there, pinning up notices around the walls, was younger than I'd thought but she looked rather tired. Her scarlet suit and gold jewellery looked like a uniform that didn't belong to her and she hadn't got round to putting on the make-up to match. When she heard me open the door she looked up and smiled.

'I can guess who you are,' she said. 'I've been wanting to meet the man who's been stealing my clients.'

I didn't know how to take that so I asked her if she liked the room.

'It's fine. In fact, compared to St Marks it's wonderful. The lights work, the loos flush and I don't have to move the jumble just to make a space for the chairs. I wish I could afford to be here permanently.'

'Why didn't you find somewhere else a bit sooner then?'

'Well, for one thing, people know where I am. I've been running my group for five years now and I get a lot of repeat business. I'm local and people like me.'

'What do you mean by repeat business? I thought the idea was for people to learn how to be thin and then go away and get a life.'

'If you don't mind me saying so, Peter – it is Peter, isn't it? that just shows how little you know about it. Of course they can't go away and get a life. Slimming is a way of life. It's not something you get fixed once, like having a tooth out. It's more like having your hair done. You have to get your highlights done regularly or you look worse than you did before you started.'

I couldn't resist smiling when she said that and I ran my fingers over my non-existent highlights. She glanced at her own immaculate blond bob in one of the mirrors and for the first time she laughed.

'OK, maybe our hairstyles sum up our attitudes. Peter, you are coming at life from a different angle to the people you're trying to help. You've got PMA instead of PMS.'

'Oh, come on, Miriam. Even I know that's sexist!'

First we form habits, then they form us

Conquer your bad habits or they'll eventually conquer you

Dr Rob Gilbert

'No, hear me out. You're thin, fit and full of enthusiasm. People with weight problems are not going to identify with you, are they? Now I've been through it all myself, and in fact my daughter's got weight problems ("so Mo was right!" I thought). I know what these people are up against and I'm here to help them fight the constant battle – because that's what it is.'

'I can see you believe in what you're doing Miriam, but I think your attitude's incredibly depressing. You make it sound like being overweight is a life sentence with no time off for good behaviour. I don't believe that. You're telling people that they've got to live lives of self-denial and abstinence forever. It's enough to make them want to go out and binge.'

'That's exactly what they do,' she said. 'From time to time. Then they come back to me and we start again. You see, I never give up on people. They know they can always come back.'

'So you agree with me that 95% of people who go on diets regain the weight they lost and often more?'

She nodded. 'I didn't know it was as high as that, but it doesn't surprise me. It's sad, I know, but that's what I tell them, "it's a battle for life" I say, "literally".'

"And what a life!" I thought. No wonder she looked so tired and depressed. Running a business based on failure might be profitable but it could hardly be exhilarating. And no wonder the daughter had rebelled. That sounded promising. I was willing to bet that the calorie police were on permanent patrol in Miriam's house.

'Anyway,' said Miriam, 'I must get on. Haven't even done my make-up yet and I've only got five minutes. It's been nice talking to you Peter. And I've got a piece of advice for you that I don't suppose you'll take, but here it is anyway. Where you're going wrong is by not giving people the kind of support they need. They're coming to you and me because they've got a big problem in their lives and you're just telling them to go out and get in touch with their personal blueprints! Many years ago, my dear, I was one of the flower power generation but we grew out of that sort of thing when we realised it didn't work. What works is giving people proper guidelines. Scales, personal weight charts, targets, calorie counters, menus, that sort of thing. Telling them to go away and learn to trust their bodies is crap. Pardon my language. But I'll leave you to find out for yourself.'

I thanked her politely and ran up the stairs. 'By the way,' she called after me, 'tell Faye her diet pack's arrived. She can pick it up on her way out tonight.'

Upstairs I tried to clear some space in the junk room. I wished I'd started earlier and I was trying to figure out if I had enough chairs when Ben and Lewis arrived carrying a pile of them.

'Mind readers!' I said. I looked sideways at Lewis, wondering whether he was going to challenge me in front of the group or keep it personal.

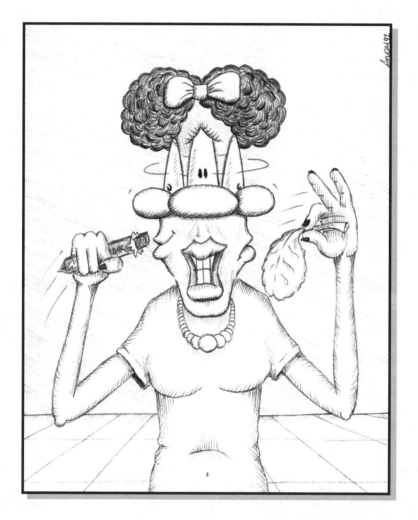

Coping With A Conventional Diet

Ben started to spread them out. 'Jane said you might need some, she was on her way out when we arrived.'

'Lovely looking girl,' said Lewis 'pity about the garlic. In my opinion women should stick to cooking it, not eating it.'

Just then Faye turned up with her friend. She pulled me to one side. 'I'm sorry about that phone call,' she said 'and I appreciate you getting back to me and explaining what you were trying to do. I'd had a bad week and I don't cope with changes very well. I knew that what I was doing wasn't working – and it was familiar. You see Pete, the thing about the other groups is they tell you exactly what to do. I suppose that's why they don't work for very long. I can see your point about taking control of your own body and working from your own blueprint, but it does take a bit more effort doesn't it? I didn't feel up to it last week to be honest.'

I stopped putting out the chairs. 'That's the trouble with the dieting industry, Faye. It implies that we are unable to manage our bodies and our eating. We have lost touch with natural responses to our physical and emotional needs. Our self acceptance and self respect are gone. People love the security of a diet because they're afraid they don't know how to eat and most diets tell you exactly what to do. My goal is to teach you how to listen to yourself, instead of having to listen to me.'

'I like listening to you. If I listened to me I'd just eat all the time,' said Faye, sadly.

'No you wouldn't, you'd eat when you were hungry, sleep when you were tired and do something exciting when you got bored…Anyway, it's about being independent again. You don't want to spend a night a week sitting in a diet group for the rest of your life, do you? Think about it Faye, you could be spending the time and money on something more exciting.' I did a quick brain-sort for something that might catch her imagination. 'You could take an evening class in belly dancing.'

That made her laugh, it did me good to hear it. 'You're kidding.'

'No I'm not,' I told her. 'I saw it on the adult education list round at the college when I was running a step class the other night. I thought I might try it, but apparently I'd be the only male!'

'Alright Pete, you've got the message across. I'm not giving up yet. Neither is Eve, are you Sweetheart?'

Her friend leaned across. 'I told Faye, she's got to give it a bit longer. We neither of us were getting on right well with some of those exercises you gave us. Personally, I can't picture things. I can hear a voice, or a tune, but you ask me to picture my front door and I can't do it. I can tell you it's green, but that's as far as it goes.'

'That's rubbish,' Faye protested, 'You have dreams, like everybody else, don't you? You see things in your dreams? Why not when you're awake?'

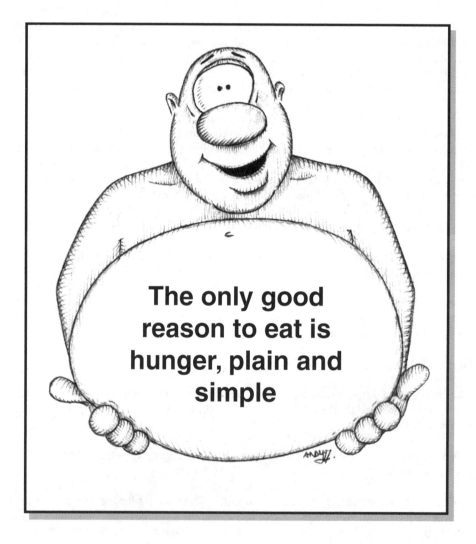

Eve thought about that for a bit. 'It's different. There are quite a lot of things I can do in my dreams that I'd love to do when I am awake. And I can tell you that looking at my front door's not top of the list. But life's not like that, is it. Anyway, I must admit that when Faye and I got together on Monday night and did the 'What Do You Want?' it worked a lot better. Plus we had a good laugh. It's a lot easier if you get somebody else to ask the questions. It might be helpful if you mentioned that in the group Pete.'

'The thing is,' I said, 'that doing the exercises with a friend works better for some people and some people prefer to do them on their own. I'm really glad you found the right way for you, Faye, but the message is, "if what you're doing doesn't work, do something different".'

'I know, I know, we're getting the message, we've got to be flexible, right? It's not easy at our age, is it Faye?'

'Those stairs are a real killer for a start' Faye replied. The two women linked arms and laughed. 'We nearly went to Miriam's just so we wouldn't have to climb the stairs. You know, sometimes I wish there was a pill you could take to keep your weight down, with no side effects and then we could spend Friday night down the pub like we used to.'

'There is, you just took one!'

'What?'

'A fat burning pill with no side effects. Walking upstairs instead of taking a lift, running for the bus, digging the garden – those are all fat burning pills.'

By this time, everybody had arrived. Lisa and Mo were late and I didn't recognise the woman they had with them. There was something odd about her but I didn't have time to give it any thought.

We were talking about including feelings in the Food Diaries and looking for patterns and Faye was giving us a blow-by-blow account of her stormy relationship with bakewell tarts when Lewis struck.

'While I'm sure we're all totally fascinated by your love affair with the cake shop' he said, 'I would like to ask Mr Motivator to explain exactly what our feelings have got to do with our weight.'

'Oh,' said Faye, who obviously had no sense of self preservation. 'I can tell you that. It's obvious: you get depressed, you eat, you get fat, you get more depressed because you're fat, and so on. Right girls?' She looked around for confirmation from the other ladies of a certain age and there was a roar of audience participation.

Keep walking and keep smiling

Tiny Tim

'I eat when I'm tired.'

'When I'm lonely.'

'Bored.'

'Frustrated.'

'Stressed.'

'Happy.'

'You see what I mean!' Faye was triumphant. 'That's why Pete's telling us to record our feelings in the diary.'

'The only good reason for eating,' I added, 'is hunger, and not just hunger at 2 or 3 on the Hunger Scale. You should be getting a good, stomach-rumbling 8 at least. If you discover from the food diary that every time you get a phone call from your ex-girlfriend, you reach for the biscuit tin, you can do something else instead.'

'Like what?' asked Eve.

'Try some breathing exercises, take a short walk, stroke the cat, light a candle, call somebody else who cheers you up. There are lots of things you can do that won't make you feel bad afterwards and won't cost anything either. Eating isn't the right way to respond to feeling bad because it's the wrong remedy for the problem.'

'It's like spoilt children.' Faye suddenly said. 'Whatever you give them in the way of toys or sweets is never enough if what they really need is love and attention. Maybe that's the reason I can never get enough food into me when I'm unhappy. How can you ever have enough of something if it's not what you really want in the first place?'

'Well, I'm sorry to disillusion you, but I'm not overweight because I'm depressed or stressed or anything else,' continued Lewis. 'I'm overweight because I have a sedentary job and I eat too much. It would be a lot more to the point if we could get some useful information from our Expert here about the balance between food and exercise. After all, we've had the lecture on calories as units of heat. What we need now is some advice on burning them up efficiently. If I want to talk about my feelings I'll go to a psychiatrist.'

'Stroppy bugger,' said Faye. 'You remind me of my son. He thinks all my problems are down to my age. 'You can laugh now.' I tell him: 'When you get to forty, you won't be able to take the beer and chips either without it showing round your waistline.' Mind you,' she added, turning round to face Lewis, 'you haven't got much of a waistline left anyway, have you?'

I suddenly remembered I was meant to be helping these people instead of sitting back and letting them entertain me.

When you eat, concentrate on the taste and texture of what you're eating

Separate eating from other activities

Remember, calories should be tasted not wasted

'Some people find there's a relationship between their feelings and their eating patterns and some people don't,' I said. 'You don't all need to tell me what you discovered, you just need to find out for yourselves. For some of you, it may be times of day, or particular activities, but you can bet there will be a pattern somewhere. And knowing it is the key to changing it. You can't change something you don't know about, can you?'

I looked directly at Ben and Lewis. 'For example, I know that some people can't watch TV unless they're into the lager and pizzas at the same time. Pity really, because they don't get half the pleasure from the food that they would if they took time to enjoy it for it's own sake.'

'I did it twice,' called Mo from the back. 'It was weird.'

'Did what twice, and why was it weird?'

'Did nothing.'

It was getting surreal. 'What?'

'Nothing while I was eating,' she said impatiently.

'Why was it weird?'

'Well, just sitting there concentrating on the food. There were a couple of nights when Lisa was out and I cooked myself supper as usual. But, sitting there just eating without the radio or the TV on, it just seemed like there was more food than I needed, I couldn't finish it.'

'And what about the next night?'

'Well, that was even stranger. I put less on the plate and sort of tarted it up a bit so it looked nice. More like I would do for customers. I don't bother with that sort of thing at home. Anyway, it was salmon and new potatoes, which is just about my favourite simple meal, and it was wonderful. Orgasmic. I didn't realise just how much I really love it.'

'But what was strange about it?'

'I didn't want any more when I'd finished. You'd think, with enjoying it so much, I'd want to keep eating and prolong the experience, wouldn't you? But, for once, I just knew when I'd had enough and I wasn't tempted to keep nibbling through the evening. It was like, I knew I'd eaten well and that was enough.'

I started clapping. 'Come on. Let's have a round of applause for Mo. That was a real success story you've just been listening to and I want you to get used to congratulating yourselves when you've done well. Don't be shy about it, it's really important.'

GOOD NEWS AND BAD NEWS

After being on a conventional diet for two weeks the rate at which you digest food can drop by 20%. That's the bad news.

The good news is that if you want to speed up your metabolism then regular physical activity will do it for you.

The last item was the hunger scale. 'How are you getting on?' I asked. I know at least two people here who thought it was a non-starter.'

Lisa and Mo were looking at each other. 'A couple of times this week' said Lisa, 'I've actually stopped and said to myself "am I hungry?" and I've had to say, "no, not really" and I do know what I feel like when I'm hungry, I can remember that far back. I'm sure it's different for everybody, but for me it's a really sharp feeling – oh, and my stomach rumbles as well. But that lunchtime I have to admit I was 3 or 4 or less on the hunger scale.'

'So what happened?'

'What do you think! I went right ahead and had lunch as usual.'

Everybody laughed.

'Well' said Eve, 'at least you stopped and thought about it, that's a start. Eating's not something I ever think about. I just do it, all the time. I've digested it before I've noticed it sometimes. I don't get a proper lunch-break so I have to just grab a bite when the phones aren't too busy.'

'So' Lewis turned to face her, 'you're one of those switchboard operators who answers with her mouth full so you can't tell whether you've dialled the right number or not.'

'I'm not just a switchboard operator, Love,' said Eve. 'I'm a Managing Director, Finance Director, Sales Director and Switchboard Operator. What do you do, when you're not being rude to women old enough to be your mother?'

'He's a computer programmer.' Ben told her. He looked like he was planning to have a few words with Lewis after the class.

'Oh, a techie.' there was every sign that Eve was about to turn on Lewis and eat him alive. 'I've always wanted to meet a real one of those. Our business is too small, we can't afford somebody like you. We have to sort our own problems out. You don't look like one though. I thought they were all thin with rows of pens in their top pockets.'

It was definitely time to close the session. 'Before you all go, I want you to keep trying with the Hunger Scale. And also concentrating more on eating. See if you can at least have one meal a day set aside for pure enjoyment. Just eating and tasting every mouthful with great pleasure. That's it for this week. Enjoy!'

Lisa stayed for the exercise class but Mo had disappeared. I grabbed Lisa at the end.

'Well, what did you think?'

'About your slimming group? Interesting. but I'm reserving judgement. By the way, it's Mo's birthday a week tomorrow. I thought we'd take her to the Sampan. Can you come?'

TAKE IT EASY

Exercise should always be comfortable regardless of your fitness level. If you can't talk or whistle at the same time, you're overdoing it. If you're hating every second and feeling totally out of breath, it's because your body isn't getting oxygen to your muscles. This isn't doing you any good.

The following Friday I looked in on Miriam again on the way up to my class. She had an even more powerful suit on and this time she'd done the face to match. Quite a difference. When she wasn't looking tired she looked tough. She looked like she was out to save the world. Or conquer it.

She smiled at me. That was scary. 'How did it go last week?' she asked.

'Fine. I gave Faye your message.'

'Thanks, I'm a teeny bit worried about Faye. She might seem quite bright and bubbly to you, but I know she gets a little bit low sometimes and that's when she binges. Her husband doesn't live at home all the time and she worries about her son a lot.'

'It sounds like grown-up children can be quite a problem,' I said. I'm not usually so bitchy but I'd had enough of Miriam telling me I didn't understand my clients.

'How would you know – about children or anything else,' muttered Miriam. Louder she said 'People are going to get awfully tired of all those stairs to your group you know. It's not really fair on the larger ladies.'

'Well maybe the really motivated ones will lose the weight just running up to my classes and the ones that come to you can just have a nice sit down and work out how many calories they can burn by counting calories.'

'I heard all of that and I'm surprised at the pair of you!' It was Mo standing in the doorway. 'Hello Miriam. How's your daughter? I haven't seen either of you since the wedding.'

'Fine thank you.'

'Shall I take some chairs up Pete?'

'Please. I'll be right with you.'

I couldn't see Lisa but the Third Woman was right behind Mo. I watched in astonishment as she picked up an enormous stack of chairs and sprinted up the stairs with them.

Miriam was still standing beside me.

'What I said was out of order, I'm sorry Peter. Oh, and I meant to ask you. Faye said you'd mentioned a fat burning pill? What's that all about? I have to tell you I'm not happy about any of these chemical aids to weight loss. From what I've read, the amphetamine based ones are addictive and the ones that are supposed to bind the fat don't work plus they all have side effects.'

'Hey Miriam this is a breakthrough – something we can actually agree on. I'm doing Fat Burning Pills in tonight's session, so why don't you ask Faye about it afterwards.'

BE A FAT BURNING MACHINE NOT A FAT STORING MACHINE

Fifteen minutes of continuous activity seems to be the time trigger that stimulates production of fat-burning enzymes. The more fat burning enzymes you have, the more fat you can burn.

But although it takes fifteen minutes to start the enzymes increasing, you are actually burning fat right from the very first step you take with the enzymes you already have.

I dashed upstairs to find that Lisa, Mo and friend had put out the chairs for me and were chatting to Ben and Lewis while the others took their seats. I couldn't remember if I'd introduced them or not. There are so many different bits to my life I sometimes forget where they overlap.

'This week,' I announced, 'I'm going to get you started on the Fat Burning Pills. We're not talking about Fen-Phen or Fat Magnets. These are free, safe and they work for everybody.'

Mo started laughing. 'Don't believe him,' she called out from the back. 'The last one I took nearly killed me!'

'That's because you overdosed instead of taking a regular low dose,' I said.

Faye joined in, 'it's walking up stairs, isn't it? You told us last week. I went to one of those Step classes once. Never again. It's like paying a fiver to get on and off a bus for fifty minutes. You might as well stay at home, put the radio on and hop on and off the bottom of the stairs.'

I caught Lewis's expression. 'Hello, Lewis, come in.'

'You can't tell us anything we don't know about fitness and training,' he said. 'We used to train five nights a week as well as Sunday afternoons and play a match every Saturday.'

'Oh so that's what it takes to burn off forty pints of lager calories is it?' asked Lisa.
'I'm sorry to say it was a lot more than that,' said Ben, 'Those were the days.'

'The secret, as usual,' I told them, 'is balance.' I pointed to the FIT principle poster I'd stuck on the wall.

'Why does it have to be so bloody boring?' said Faye.

'Why does it have to hurt so much?' added Mo.

'If it's boring you're doing the wrong exercise for you and if it hurts you're doing too much or for too long. Obviously if you've been sedentary for a while you've got to work up to it gradually. Forget what you've heard about going for the burn. It's rubbish.' Looking around, I could see everybody looking sceptical at that. But I certainly had their attention.

'You don't believe me' I continued, 'but you'd all really like to, wouldn't you? I'm not telling you anything you don't know already, but I'm asking you to take it seriously for once. It's this simple. As you become more active, you become fitter. I know that not everybody has a job like mine and works in a building with no lift. I know that some of you used to be a lot more active than you are now — and I know you can't necessarily go back to your old lifestyles again. Things change and you have to try and change your patterns of eating and exercising to match your new lifestyles. It's like dieting, you have to find the level that's right for you.'

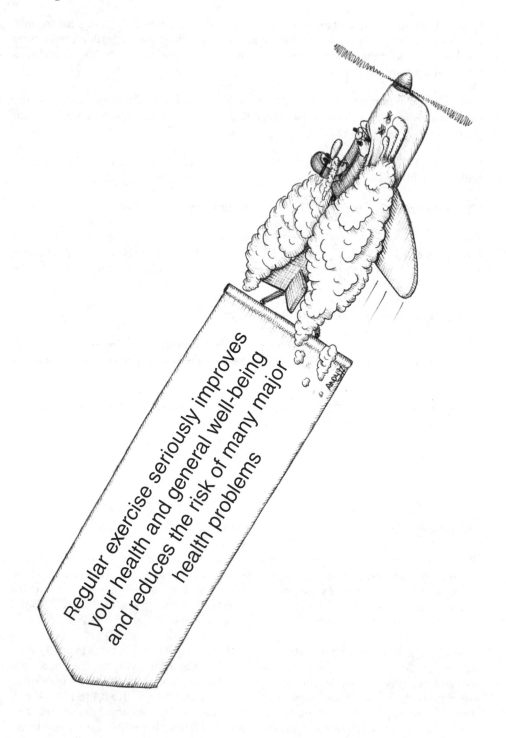

Regular exercise seriously improves your health and general well-being and reduces the risk of many major health problems

'But what exactly does that mean?' asked Ben. 'Obviously Faye and I aren't going to need identical fitness programmes ...'

'I don't know,' said Faye, 'maybe if we do the same workout I could drink eight pints and sink a curry afterwards – in fact, me and the girls could join you for the odd night out ...'

'Stop winding him up Faye.' I had a sudden flashback to my days as a PE teacher. I remembered thinking how much easier it would be to work with adults than it was with adolescents. It just shows, doesn't it, how wrong I was.

Ben was determined to make his point. 'All I want to ask Pete is how we're going to know whether we're getting our exercise programme right or not?'

'By the results you get, basically. And I'm not talking about pounds and ounces. When you start to feel and look better you'll know you're getting it right. If you start to look thinner but you're feeling terrible' I couldn't stop myself catching Lisa's eye but I looked away again quickly, 'you're not getting it right. Feelings and results have to go together.'

'The exercise you do has five components: how often you do it, at what sort of level, how long you do it for and what is most exciting for you.' Everybody was giggling. Faye and friends were the most raucous. 'And, lastly,' I said, 'it's important to do it regularly.'

It was ages before I could make myself heard again. I decided to re-word that part of the programme for the next group. When they had all calmed down, we spent some time going through the different ways of working out what you need to do. Then Faye started off on her own agenda again. 'I've heard that regular exercise helps prevent osteoporosis? My Mum's crippled with it.'

Ben and Lewis had been quite well behaved so far, but they could spot a Women's Issue a mile away. They were sighing loudly and looking at each other, so I set the record straight.

'Its not just osteoporosis. Regular exercise also reduces the risk of heart disease, strokes, diabetes, arthritis, high blood pressure, cancer, back pain and stress related illnesses. What's more, it raises your body temperature and gives you more energy. I think you'll agree there's something for everybody there.'

'So you save money on thermal underwear, hospital bills and bus fares – does it make you rich and famous as well?' asked Mo.

'You're not going to be rich and famous unless you do a lot of it,' said her friend, who was sitting beside her.

I got the feeling I was preaching to the converted so I thought it would be a good idea to send them all home with a Fat Jar.

'I've already got a Fat Jar,' said Faye, 'it's me.'

THE BENEFITS OF EXERCISE

The benefits of exercise, apart from making you slimmer, are almost endless.

Exercise reduces:

Arthritis

Back pain

Cancer

Diabetes

Fatty deposits in arteries

Heart disease

High blood pressure

Osteoporosis

Stress and tension

Strokes

'Well then it's time you got a different one. One you can leave on the table when you go out.' I produced an empty coffee jar and seven 5p pieces. 'This is a week's supply – for now. You'll be gradually increasing the dose till you find the right level. What you're starting to work on is changing your own chemistry. Fat people store glucose as fat whereas fit people store it as glycogen which is easier to use. People who are overweight have different fat cells. It's the enzymes in the fat cells that convert food into stored fat. These enzymes are especially active in fat people.

By increasing your exercise levels you can actually decrease the level of your fat storing enzymes. By simply cutting back on what you eat, you trigger the body's instinctive reaction against starvation which is to try to store more fat. And whatever weight you do succeed in losing, you're very likely to regain it, plus a bit extra in the form of fat, as soon as you stop dieting.

And there's another thing you change by exercising. When fit people exercise, the PH level of their blood changes and directly decreases their feelings of hunger.'

'So the more you exercise, the less hungry you get? Pull the other one.' Faye was open-mouthed with disbelief.

'You will feel as hungry as you need to be. The exercise will make your real hunger feelings kick in. What you won't get is the pseudo-hunger that springs from boredom or unhappiness or whatever. So you'll know when you need to eat, but you won't get false readings any more. So make a start with these Fat Burning Pills. Like I said, they're nothing short of a miracle. No side effects, no prescription, no cost, no failures. There are just two things you have to remember. Put them in the jar instead of swallowing them and each one takes between ten and fifteen minutes to work. What they actually do is make your fat storage system less efficient. Bad if you live in a famine-stricken part of the world. Good if you live in snack city.'

Mo raised her hand. 'What sort of exercise does one pill consist of? And what about people like Lisa? She exercises already. What difference is it going to make to her?'

'To start with I want you all to just try and add one pill per day to whatever your normal routine happens to be. Just make sure there are at least five in the jar at the end of the week. For now, the only exercise that counts is brisk walking. And those of you who work out anyway, just add the fifteen minutes of brisk walking into your routine.'

'I always knew there was a really good reason to go on to a club after dinner. My name's Chris, by the way,' said Lisa's friend.

'Isn't it funny,' added Lisa, 'how good you feel after you've been dancing and how awful you feel when you've done a workout. And yet, when you think about it, a workout on the dance floor can be just as energetic as in the gym.'

'We don't all have such a wonderful social life,' said Faye, 'I'm more likely to be doing the washing up and ironing than going dancing after dinner.'

Exercise increases:

Appetite control

Efficiency of the digestive system

Energy

Delivery of nutrients to the body

Secretion of endorphins which act as relaxants

Ability to sleep well

'Any activity's better than just sitting in front of the box.' I was handing out fat jars and 5p pieces. 'And you've got a good point Lisa. Exercise should make you feel good as well as making you stronger and reducing your risk of all sorts of diseases. You've finally admitted that there's at least one form of exercise you get some fun out of. Why not quit the gym and spend more time on the dance floor? You'll get more benefit because you'll put more effort into it and you'll be less likely to drop out.'

Lisa looked thoughtful.

'What do we do with the 5p pieces?' Asked Lewis.

'Save them up till the end of all the sessions and we'll have a party. Oh, and speaking of parties, I want you to come to the group registering at least 8 or 9, if not 10 on the Hunger Scale next week. Don't eat before you come, I'm going to feed you all. Any questions?'

Afterwards Mo disappeared quite quickly with Chris. I thought Lisa would stay on for the aerobics as usual but she was already on her way out. She paused to remind me about the birthday party at the Chinese the following night.

Lewis and Ben overheard us and Lewis moved right in and put his arm round Lisa who flinched, very slightly. 'Are we invited? After all, if we're going to share our problems for the next few Friday nights maybe we should help you celebrate Mo's birthday. All in the interests of bonding and solidarity of course.'

Lisa looked uncertain. 'Oh, why not, the more the merrier. It's at the Sampan, you know, just along from the Duke's Head.'

'We know it,' said Ben, 'we must be some of their best customers. I'm surprised we haven't seen you there before.'

Lisa looked at him. 'I suspect you tend to eat after closing time so we've probably never overlapped. You're welcome to join us tomorrow, but we're meeting at 8 and we're not going to wait for you if you get stuck in the pub first.'

I was walking to the restaurant the following night when a car pulled up alongside. It was Lewis in a new, silver BMW. There didn't seem to be much point since we were almost at the Sampan but I thought if I'd got to work with him for a few more slimming sessions we might as well try to get along. 'Where's Ben?' I asked as I sank into the upholstery. It had one of those seat belts that comes up to meet you. I think they're creepy.

'Oh, he's taking his fat pill for the day, and I think he's going to take another one after the meal. At least he is if I have anything to do with it, I thought I might offer Lisa a lift. Very pretty that girl, even if she is a bit skinny.'

'Lisa's a good friend of mine. Respect her or leave her alone.'

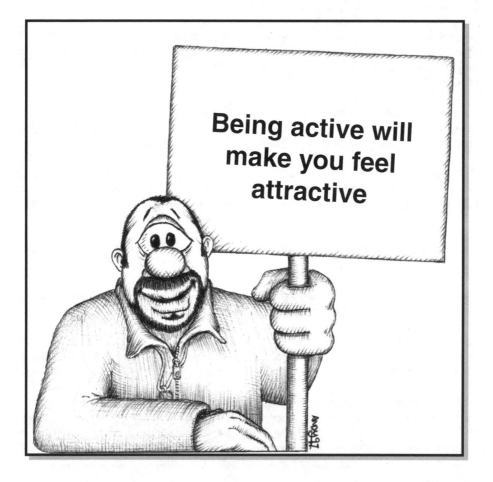

He laughed and then started cursing when he couldn't park right outside the Chinese. I could have told him it was impossible mid-evening on a Saturday but I thought he might as well find out for himself. 'I'll hop out here' I said. 'You'll probably have to go to the multi-story. We'll keep a place for you.'

I stepped through the door to find Lisa already there, fair and fragile as ever. She looked worried. I took the seat next to her and gave her a hug. 'What's the matter?'

'Mo was going to collect Chris. She should be here by now.'

'Was she in the car?'

'No, she decided to walk, like me. We're both taking the pills — you ought to be proud of us!'

Before I could answer some of the others arrived, then, shortly afterwards, Ben came in. Conversation stopped. It was the first time I'd seen him in a suit and he reminded me of Wesley Snipes. It seemed likely that none of the other men would get much attention for the rest of the evening, and I wondered how Lewis would feel about being upstaged. Ben sat down on the other side of Lisa and just as the menus were being handed round Mo, Chris and Lewis turned up together.

Poor Mo was completely dwarfed by her companions and she looked glamorous but stressed. I waved at her to come and sit by me while we made our choices. Every time the waiter hovered with a pen and pad Lisa said she wasn't ready. 'It all looks wonderful,' she said. Then she suddenly announced that she wasn't hungry because she'd eaten before she came out.

'No you didn't,' said Mo.

'Yes I did – you left before me, remember? I just felt I wouldn't last till we got to the restaurant so I had a sandwich after you'd gone. Where have you been anyway? I thought you'd got lost?' said Lisa.

I was starting to have a bad feeling about this party. Suddenly I couldn't concentrate on the menu either. 'Let's order some champagne ... it's my treat.' When it arrived I noticed Lisa and Ben cover their glasses as the waiter moved around the table.

I looked at Ben inquiringly, 'You're not driving are you?'

He laughed 'It isn't that, I just haven't had time to eat much today and it's a really bad idea to drink on an empty stomach. Mind you, I'm definitely up to 9 on the hunger scale.'

'Yes, we can all hear that,' Lewis told him.

Lisa looked at Ben with interest. She'd never had much in common with him when they'd met at my place in the past. She didn't like rugby or lager even before she became so diet conscious. It was almost as if she thought he was joining the human race at last.

Be bold and mighty forces will come to your aid

Basil King

'I thought you were looking slimmer,' she said.

Ben looked pleased. 'You noticed? I lost six pounds in the last month,' he said.

He had everybody's attention. 'How?' said Lisa? 'Come on, share the secret, I've never managed to lose that much in a month. That must have been before you even joined the group. Maybe you can give me some advice.'

I was getting annoyed. 'Is anybody going to order some food? Or are you all going to sit around for the next two hours discussing what you shouldn't eat? In case you'd forgotten, the slimming class was last night. Tonight is Mo's birthday and I think she should choose what we get to talk about.'

'Alright,' Mo raised her glass. 'Happy Birthday to Me. We're not going to talk about food, we're going to eat it. And we can dance it off afterwards. Let's go to Sols, they stay open way late, and we can walk there.'

Chapter 5

Thinking And Eating

I suppose you could say that Mo's birthday party was a success. I wasn't entirely sure that Mo enjoyed it the way she used to enjoy parties in the old days, even though clubbing afterwards was her idea. It was Lisa who seemed to have the best time at Sols. I was watching her dancing with Ben and thinking it was a pity she didn't like my classes as much as she loved being on the dance floor. After all, what was the difference? Music and lots of fancy footwork. And in the gym she'd be wearing trainers; those high heels might be a shoe fetishist's dream, but I couldn't imagine how she could keep going on them for hours. In fact, at one point when she came back up to the bar, where I was sitting watching the action I said to her 'You could twist an ankle in those. If you want to take them off, I'll look after them for you.'

She gave me a very funny look. 'Not you as well.' Then she laughed and was gone again. The next thing I knew, Mo turned up on the bar stool next to mine. She waved at the barman to bring her another beer and looked at me sideways. 'It's my birthday and if I want to have a couple of beers, I will. Besides, I'm sure I'm dancing it off.'

'Hey I didn't even say anything! But if you want me to start being picky, I could point out that your birthday finished a couple of hours ago. I thought you were dancing with Lewis. Where is he?'

'Between you and me, I got the impression that he really wanted to be with Lisa, it's just that Ben got there first. You've heard the story of my life often enough. Especially since I met Lisa. My Mother used to say, "If you want to get on, find yourself an ugly friend", And why didn't I listen to my mother? Slim, blonde flatmates are such bad news if you happen to be a little brown mouse.'

I looked at Mo. It was weeks since her hair had been mousy. I don't quite know what colour I'd describe it as, sort of dark raspberry I think. It suited her, although she looked rather pale and she was probably a bit too old to be a Goth.

'Just for the record, you're not mousy. You are one of those women who look as good as you feel and just recently you've been glowing. What happened tonight – and why are you on your own?'

'I'm not, it just feels like it. Anyway, what about you? Didn't you have a mysterious date at a wine bar a couple of weeks ago? Why isn't she here tonight?'

'The lady I met that night is away on business.' I shrugged. "At least, that's what she told me", I thought, but I wasn't going to air my doubts out loud.

A path with no obstacles goes nowhere

So be prepared for challenging times and you will find yourself overcoming them

'Sounds like we're both in the same boat.' She was picking sadly at the peanuts, one at a time. Seeing me look at her hand, she stopped, halfway to her mouth. 'How many have I eaten?'

'Why don't you eat the rest – and enjoy them?'

'Enjoy them! I wouldn't even have noticed them if you hadn't looked at me like that. Oh, God, that's so typical. What am I going to do? I've just had a Chinese meal, and toffee bananas. I'm stuffed and yet I'm still eating peanuts.'

'Stop it. One little lapse doesn't matter. I don't know what's bugging you tonight, but something is. Come on, I'll dance with you, it's a better way of taking your mind off your troubles than eating peanuts. Let's see just how good we can feel. Where's your friend Chris by the way? I'd like to meet her.'

Mo scanned the floor. It was packed now. Hard to see who was who. Suddenly she laughed. 'Oh, no, I don't believe it. Chris is dancing with Lewis. He's going to be so upset. I'll rescue him.'

It was at that point I decided to leave them all to it and walk home. I woke up next morning to hear the phone ringing and reached out to grab it. Mo was at the other end.

'What happened to you last night? When I got back to the bar you were gone. I was going to introduce you to Chris. Are you alright?'

Mo was always one to worry about other people. Lisa was a lovely person, but very often she couldn't see beyond her own problems. 'I'm fine, I just felt like a spare whatsit at a wedding.'

'Well, you know you wanted to meet Chris? Why not come round and have breakfast with us.'

I didn't take much persuading. My kitchen was halfway through being renovated and I couldn't do much more than make a cup of tea in it. The idea of a proper breakfast was very appealing.

Half an hour later, I was knocking at their door. I could smell the coffee even before Mo let me in. She hugged me and pulled me down the stairs. The kitchen seemed to be full of people but I realised it was only Lisa and a tall man in jeans and a black T shirt. He had his back to me and he was bending over the cooker. The previous evening flashed through my head. "Who took who home?" I thought.

I could see it wasn't Ben, he's pretty distinctive from any angle. Lewis? I hoped not. 'Hi,' I said and waited. The man turned round and he certainly wasn't Lewis. He looked familiar, but I couldn't place him. He smiled and wiped his hand on a tea towel before holding it out to me.

'Chris?'

My philosophy is that, not only are you responsible for your life, but doing the best at this moment puts you in the best place for the next moment

Oprah Winfrey

'Well done.' A lot of people don't believe what they see. We never got a chance to talk last night, did we?' There was a slight New York accent. Like just a trace of Lloyd Grossman.

I sat down and grabbed the coffee pot. 'Now I see why Mo thought there might be trouble if you danced with Lewis. How do you get away with the cross-dressing, and why?'

'It's my job. Times are tough at the moment, there are too many people doing what I do. I needed to run some street trials if you know what I mean.'

'No, actually, I haven't got a clue. And tell me, how did you meet Mo?' Another thought occurred to me.

I couldn't quite believe it. 'Mo, is this...'

'The man, of course!' Lisa was delighted to be the one to break the news. 'You know last time we talked even I hadn't met him. Chris is Mo's big secret.'

He was certainly big. Over six foot, with a trace of a beard. How could I ever have mistaken him for a woman?

'We look like Little and Large, don't we?' Mo was absolutely glowing and she was wearing make-up and a dress on a Sunday morning.

'What we look like doesn't matter. It's how we feel about each other that counts.' Chris looked back over his shoulder to smile at her.

'Would you like me and Lisa to go out for breakfast and leave you two alone?' I wasn't sure how much of this sort of thing I could stand first thing on Sunday morning.

'Don't be silly. Chris is making porridge.'

He looked round again. 'I used to be a chef before I went into the entertainment business. Porridge, fruit and granary toast isn't my idea of breakfast but it's all Mo and Lisa will allow.'

It smelt wonderful. I went over and sniffed. 'Is this healthy breakfast because of me?'

'Don't kid yourself. It was Mo's idea. She's trying to make up for last night.' Lisa wasn't looking her best, she was wearing black jeans and her face was as grey as her elegant mohair top. Maybe it was the contrast with Mo who was glowing. 'Anyway,' she added, 'I don't see why Chris has to ruin one of my saucepans. You can make porridge in a microwave.'

'Not in yours,' said Chris, 'I couldn't get a beep out of it and it's full of aspirins anyway.'

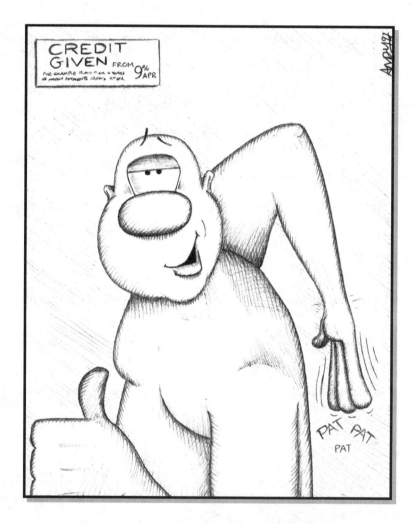

Take Responsibility For Tracking Your Triumphs

'Honestly Lisa, you know it stopped working ages ago.' Mo opened the microwave door and looked inside then slammed it in annoyance. 'You started using it as a medicine cabinet because you never cook anything anyway so you didn't miss it. If you're not on some raw energy diet where you just eat a pile of celery and carrots, you're ordering in the greasiest takeaway in the delivery area.'

'I don't know what you're trying to prove, Mo. It wasn't me who had pudding at the Sampan yesterday' said Lisa, virtuously.

'You know, I really hate it when everybody starts telling me what I'm doing wrong. As if I didn't know. And I still don't think last night was that bad. OK, a pudding and a few peanuts. Otherwise I had the same as everybody else.'

'And half a bottle of champagne, and most of the prawn crackers.'

'If I were you, Lisa, I'd shut up now before you really annoy me and I tell everybody what you did before you got to the Sampan.'

'That's ENOUGH. Mo and Lisa, please stop this right now or I'm going to suggest Pete and I head out to the greasy spoon and leave you two to eat the healthy stuff between you.'

I looked at Chris with admiration. "Very assertive", I thought. I said, 'I think we'd better stay in and help them eat it. If they pig out at breakfast, after last night, they'll be feeling so bad by teatime they'll be unbearable.'

'I usually skip breakfast altogether when I've had a big dinner,' said Lisa.

'So do you have a big lunch then?'

'No, of course not, sometimes I can distract myself so I miss out lunch as well.'

'Teatime?'

'Oh, well, you know how it is with me and chocolate bars in the afternoon. What is it about afternoons anyway? It must be a pretty common phenomenon or afternoon tea wouldn't have been invented.'

'The best way to avoid four o' clock munchies is to have breakfast and lunch. There are even diets that say you shouldn't eat anything after five.'

'Whoever thought of that one can't possibly have ever had a social life,' said Chris. 'I'm accustomed to eating late. When I was a chef, we always used to have something to eat and wind down with a glass of wine after last orders and now, I can't eat until after the show. It doesn't matter as long as you get some exercise afterwards. Going to a club – as long as you dance of course – walking home, and there are others ways of burning off the fat late at night.'

THE PLEASURE OF ACHIEVING

Take a moment to really think about all the pleasure you would gain from being slimmer

What will it be like to be slimmer and healthier?

What will you feel like?

What will you look like?

Think about it...

Mo had that look on her face again, so I joined in quickly. 'That's great for your lifestyle. But if you have to be on the train at the crack of dawn, you can't dance the night away and have breakfast at lunchtime.'

'No, but you can adapt the basic principle,' said Chris. 'I keep telling Mo, she could go for a walk after dinner, take time to think about the day, plan for tomorrow. Anything in fact, except be a couch potato in front of the bloody TV.'

I was curious. 'You know a lot about this, don't you? You don't look overweight to me and I'm asking myself why you're coming to the classes.'

'Cross-dressing always makes you look fatter than you are. I can't afford to carry any extra weight at all and I've actually gained a few pounds since I've been walking out with Mo. Mainly because we haven't been walking out much, we've been staying in.'

'I thought that sort of staying in was pretty good for using calories,' said Lisa.

'Well, it's probably got to do with more wining and dining and less clubbing to be truthful. But, if you really want to know, coming to the groups was partly for me and partly to give Mo some encouragement.'

Lisa was indignant. 'It was my idea to get Mo along to the aerobics and the weight control classes. I was going along with her anyway.'

'That was what worried me.' Chris whispered to me. Aloud, he said, 'OK, let's set the table, this is ready.' He picked up a coffee jar with 5p pieces in the bottom of it. There was another one beside it with just one coin inside. 'What are you saving up for? A ten-year subscription to "Weakly Dieting", knowing you two.'

'It's the fat jar, remember?'

'Oh, right, I forgot about that. Hey, there are three 15 minute walks' worth of fat in these already and you only started it on Friday.'

'That one's mine,' said Lisa. 'I walked home Friday, and yesterday I walked to the Mall and then to the restaurant in the evening, that's a good twenty minutes. Three lumps of fat. Easy.'

'So that was easy for you? And how easy is it going to be for you to take a brisk walk every day? I don't know just how many chances you will get to fit more brisk walking into your working routine, or how much better it's going to make you feel?'

She looked up and smiled. 'Actually, I can see myself walking a lot more. I'm all set up for it, I've got the trainers, I can keep my shoes at work and I can listen to something motivational on my Walkman. But, you know what? I still can't believe that if it's not painful it can really be doing me that much good. How long before I get to see the difference?'

The real secret of success is enthusiasm

Walter Chrysler

'You'll feel a difference, if there's going to be one, long before you see it. Your clothes won't be tight, you'll know when you're hungry and you'll feel restless if you sit still for too long.'

'What do you mean, "if there's going to be one?". I don't like the sound of that.'

'He means you don't have much more to lose,' said Chris. 'Take my advice, I see plenty of dancers who are way too thin. Don't let it happen to you Lisa. You look wonderful as you are. In fact you could gain a couple of pounds and that would look good too.'

I noticed, smugly, that sophisticated Chris had managed to annoy both Mo and Lisa in one go. I enjoyed the moment briefly and then set about repairing the situation.

'It's back to the blueprint,' I reminded them. 'Not everybody was meant to look like everybody else and there's a wide range of sizes and shapes. Your body knows what size you were meant to be and when you start trusting yourself again, that's how you'll look. Not everybody is designed to be skinny but, don't worry Mo, nobody was designed to be fat.'

'Well, the jar with only one 5p in is mine, but at least I've made a start. I had a walk yesterday to celebrate my birthday, I thought I'd start this year the way I mean to go on,' said Mo, 'I'm going to take another walk today. And, I admit it, it's easy.'

Lisa paused with a spoonful halfway to her mouth. 'Exercise or not, it still doesn't feel right, sitting down to a breakfast after last night.'

'Why don't you stop worrying about last night and thinking about today?' I suggested. 'If you both spent more time in the present and future, instead of gearing what you eat to what you ate yesterday, you might actually enjoy it. You might even break this "starve now and stuff later because I can't help it" pattern. The past is the past. Ask yourself, "what am I going to do and eat today that I'll enjoy and might even do me a bit of good?".'

Mo was looking at her bowl in desperation. There was longing in her eyes, but I knew she was silently listing everything she'd eaten the night before. 'We've had this argument before,' she said. 'Things that are good for you aren't that compelling.'

'Might I make a comment?' asked Chris. He was already on the toast. 'I couldn't help noticing, Lisa, that you hardly ate anything last night anyway.'

'Not at the restaurant,' Mo said quietly. Lisa looked daggers at her.

Chris continued, 'and as for you Mo, darling, I know you had more than you meant to, but...'

Mo leaned on his shoulder 'It wasn't my fault, I was feeling a bit down because we couldn't, you know, dance together. It was my birthday and I felt like a wallflower.'

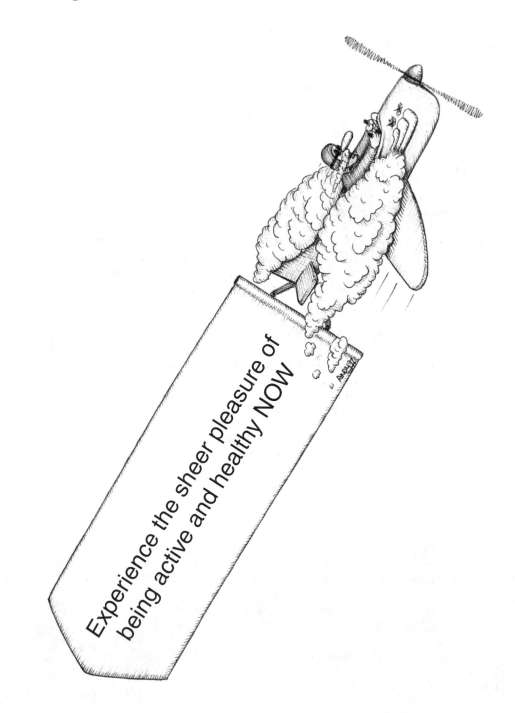

Experience the sheer pleasure of being active and healthy NOW

Chris put his hand under her chin and looked at her. 'Whatever you ate, Honey, you didn't have much after midnight. And now it's midday. That's twelve hours later! You were dancing, even if it wasn't with me. We walked home, we...'

I intervened, quickly, 'Chris is right. My professional advice is to enjoy breakfast, it's one meal where you can eat a bit more and then burn it off quite easily. How much exercise do you take on a normal Sunday by the way?'

'The whole point of Sunday is to be inactive,' said Mo. 'I work bloody hard all week and my main activity on Sunday used to be brunch followed by dinner. Unless I'm going home of course. Then I skip the brunch because I get lunch, followed by tea three hours later. Since this dieting started I can't do any of that any more so my sources of pleasure are down to reading the papers, shopping, cleaning, watching a video...'

'It's all a bit negative, when you think about it, isn't it?' Lisa pointed out. 'It's, like, our idea of fun on our day off is not doing anything special. Maybe it would be just as relaxing to actually go out and do something.'

I knew that was quite unusual for Lisa. She spent most of her life trying to avoid problems rather than actively going out to have fun. Something was changing. 'Well,' I said, 'why not break the habits of a lifetime right now? Come out with me and we'll do something exciting.'

'What would I be letting myself in for? And how much am I going to enjoy it?' asked Lisa. 'I distinctly remember you giving us that lecture about pleasure and pain last week.'

Chris looked interested. 'Oh really?'

I was beginning to like him. 'I don't know what you had in mind, but my pleasure and pain principle is about real life and food and motivation. It's just that this constant bloody preoccupation with losing weight and failing to do it ...'

'Which you make money out of.' Mo reminded me.

'You're always saying that. The difference is that, unlike most of the multi-million pound diet industry, I am interested in people cracking the problem and getting on with something more positive. I only want to see my clients one time around. Present company excepted. I don't want to run a lonely hearts club like Miriam does, for the overweight and under-motivated. Tell me this, what comes to mind when you think of the word "diet"?'

'Pain' said Lisa and Mo together.

'Right. The reason most diets fail is simply because people associate them with pain. Not that that's surprising. A lot of them are painful. And most people associate the other big weight-loss factor with pain as well.'

THINK BEFORE YOU EAT

Different events, feelings, times and trigger situations can make you feel like eating, regardless of whether you're really hungry

So if you are triggered to eat for any reason apart from hunger –

DO SOMETHING ELSE!

'Exercise, I suppose you mean.'

'Yes, exercise. Now I know that eating the right amount of good food and exercising regularly isn't painful.'

'You're weird.'

'I'm not bloody weird. It's what human beings were designed to do. Be active. Sitting around all day is exactly what we weren't designed for so if you do too much of it your whole system gets out of balance. Taking some exercise is fun, it feels good. In fact, once you've got into the habit of it you won't want to live your life any other way. All I'm trying to do is get people to realise the pain they're causing themselves by eating too much crappy food and letting their muscles waste away. I want to get them to experience the sheer pleasure of the other lifestyle.'

'The good old endorphin rush. Free, organically produced, legal chemicals,' said Chris.

'Great,' said Lisa. 'So that's it, is it? You've just given away the magic formula, so now we don't need to turn up for the next six Friday nights. We can just stay at home and repeat the mantra: "press-ups mean pleasure and puddings mean pain", and we've cracked it! Hey we can save ourselves a fortune and have fun on Fridays as well!'

'Better not tell Miriam you know the Secret,' said Mo. 'She might take a contract out on you in case it gets about and she goes out of business.'

Chris was laughing. 'It sounds like a blinding flash of the obvious to me. Does anybody want any more toast? How does it feel to have some breakfast inside you, ladies?'

'Wicked,' said Mo, looking at him through her eyelashes. 'I feel I'm going to have to pay for it somehow.'

'Oh,' said Chris, 'we're back to pleasure and pain, are we? I've got a feeling that it's not quite what Pete had in mind. Let's get this washing up done. It's a warm-up exercise for the exhilarating activity that's to come.'

'What I had in mind,' I told them, 'was a bike ride along the tow path and then back via that new pizza place you were talking about last night.'

'Exhilarating! Exhausting, more like!' exclaimed Mo. 'What do you think I am? Fit or something? That's a four mile round trip, I swear it is. Anyway, I haven't ridden my bike since last summer, and Lisa hasn't even got one.'

'We're going to hire them. We can rent helmets as well. It's a beautiful day, just go for it.'

Think Before You Eat

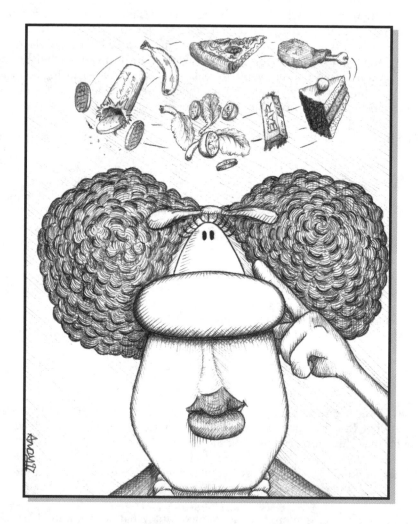

What Would Feel Good In My Stomach?

Of course, like everything always is, it was easier said than done. Getting the three of them washed up, organised and out of the house was like pulling teeth once inertia had set in. I couldn't have done it at all without some help from Chris. Admittedly, he did tell Lisa he could see the fat building up on her thighs as she was sitting in the chair. It was a little harsh, but it got her moving.

Later, as we sat over our pizza, I asked the question, 'Well, exhilarated, or exhausted?'

'Both,' said Mo, 'but the overall feeling is good. I wouldn't actually mind feeling like this more often.'

'It beats the usual Sunday "sludge" effect,' added Lisa. 'Don't we sound virtuous? You know, I might get myself a bike. I haven't ridden one since I was at school. I wouldn't mind one of those flashy hybrid things, you know, with lots of gears, like a mountain bike. But the helmet doesn't do a thing for my hair.'

'I'm sure you can get designer helmets.' Chris told her. 'You could look like one of the cast of Starlight Express. Dressing for exercise is really fashionable.'

Mo was looking relaxed. 'I don't feel as tired as I usually do on a Sunday, funny, considering I've taken about ten times the usual amount of exercise. Can I put loads of 5ps in the Fat Jar?'

'Nice try,' I said, 'but only 15 minutes of brisk walking counts. So you can put one in when you get home, provided you don't cheat and catch the bus. By the way, I need to ask a favour. My kitchen's still out of action. Can I come over on Thursday and prepare the food I'm taking to the group next Friday?'

Lisa smiled. 'No problem – just so long as you cook dinner for us at the same time.'

When Mo let me into the flat the following Thursday, I could tell by the old track suit she was wearing that Chris wasn't there.

'Where's Chris?' I asked as we went downstairs.

'Working,' said Mo, gloomily. 'He might not be able to make the group on Friday by the way. He's doing a matinee. Anyway, he doesn't really need to. He's already lost all the weight he wanted to, I think he's just coming to encourage me. Basically, he just cut out the late night kebabs, the afternoon Mars bars, and started walking to work and that was it! Seven pounds gone in a month. It's just not fair.'

'Chris was pretty fit before he even started, wasn't he? There's a lot of evidence that suggests it's a good idea to get fit before you go on a diet. A well-exercised body responds more quickly and with less muscle loss to the stress of dieting.'

'Oh, terrific. Pete, you are so good at making me feel wonderful,' said Mo. 'Talk about chicken and egg. That piece of information is about as encouraging as that thing you told me about how dieting slows down your metabolic rate. It's a real no-win situation as far as I can see.'

Before you eat, ask yourself:

How hungry am I?

What will feel good in my stomach?

How will this food make me feel after I've eaten it?

I went into the kitchen sideways, so I could get my carrier bags through the door. 'How's your exercise programme going?'

'Well, I'm trying a few new things.' Lisa took one of the bags and started emptying it. 'Last night, we decided to go for a jog round the park, didn't we, Mo?'

She nodded. 'It was Chris's idea, just because he doesn't do a show on Wednesdays he has all this spare energy and he thinks other people do as well.'

'Well, anyway,' Lisa went on, 'I usually just go to the club when I want to workout.' 'Which you don't, want to I mean,' Mo reminded her. 'You usually whinge about it.'

'Alright, I know, but jogging's dangerous.'

'I can see that. All those old men walking their dogs – you could give them heart attacks if you wear that outfit you came to last Friday's class in. Or you might trample someone underfoot.'

'I might be attacked, then you'd be sorry for being so cynical,' said Lisa. 'Anyway, we were jogging along together the three of us, chatting. Like you said, it's the right level of exercise if you can hold a conversation. After a while I noticed I was on my own, believe it or not, I actually outran Chris!'

'That's only because he was waiting for me,' said Mo. 'I had a stitch.'

'Don't give me any credit, will you. Anyway, I carried on and after a few minutes, I heard somebody behind me and I thought it was Chris. I realised you might have got left behind Mo. '

'Thanks for waiting then.' Mo looked like she was settling into a depression for the evening.

'I didn't look over my shoulder, I just started chatting to him and after a couple more minutes, he said, "Well, it's been nice talking to you, but I must get on," and he ran past me. It wasn't Chris at all. Just think, I could have been talking to anybody.'

'Well, if it was the mad rapist, he obviously didn't rate your bum from behind,' said Mo bitterly.

'Did you enjoy it?' I asked them as I sliced up the celery.

'I hated it.' Mo put her arms on the table and lay her head on them. Suddenly, she looked up. 'Tell me, Pete, which did me more good? That twenty minute jog, or the day we spent on the bikes on Sunday?'

'The one you enjoyed the most of course. If you felt uncomfortable when you were jogging, the chances are you were working too hard. In fact, if you're feeling any pain, like stitch for example, your body's telling you something. Pain's a safety mechanism. Like putting your hand on this pan without an oven glove. If you do it by accident, you get an immediate signal to stop. Comfortable, regular activity is the key. When

HUNGER PANGS

How do you know just where you are on the hunger scale? And how do you know if you're feeling hungry? Well, if you're not sure, you're probably not.

Signs of Hunger

- Smelling or tasting a food you want when it's not there
- Knowing exactly what you want to eat
- Empty feelings in the stomach
- Sharp but not unpleasant sensation in the stomach accompanied by rumbling
- Loss of energy
- Irritability
- Light-headedness
- Slightly nauseous headache accompanied by desire to eat
- Sudden fall in motivation for the task in hand
- Inability to think about anything but food

you diet, you can lose weight but still have the chemistry of a fat person. When you start including steady, enjoyable activity in your life, your body becomes more adept at burning fat always. Your muscles become more toned so that they develop more of the enzymes that burn fat and then, if you start eating more again that will probably be fine. Your body will actually need it.'

Lisa got the can opener and started on the tins of kidney beans and tuna. 'Actually, I must admit, I felt pretty good after that run. Now the nights are lighter I might do that instead of the gym, it's nice down there by the river.'

'It's like every other form of exercise, if you don't enjoy it for it's own sake, you're not going to keep it up. Remember just after Christmas, Lisa? You were coming to the gym five times a week and that's when you...' I realised I was about to be tactless and stopped, but it was too late.

'Alright, I remember. How could I forget. It's my New Year ritual. I always start January with a new resolution to be fitter and thinner. It's your idea Pete. It's what you sell, remember? Don't give me a hard time for following your advice.'

'All I'm saying is that I know so many people who start like that. They know that exercise is going to hurt. They know they're going to hate it. And the way they go about it, sure it becomes a self-fulfilling prophecy. Instead of wiping yourself out a couple of times a week, why not try a little every day, find out when you start to enjoy it, because there's always a point when you will. Listen to your body, breath deeply but don't get completely out of breath. Remember, you're not trying to burn loads of calories, you're training your body to burn fat and this is done at a comfortable level. Let your body adjust in its own time.'

Lisa patted my arm. 'Save the lecture for tomorrow. I'm hungry. At least nine on the scale.'

'How do you know when you're hungry?' I asked her.

'I get this feeling, not a pain exactly, but like, my stomach is eating itself. It rumbles as well.'

It did.

'I usually eat before I get to this stage, I haven't felt like this for ages. I suppose everybody feels it differently.'

'When I'm really hungry,' Mo told us, 'I get a bit light-headed and I can smell food two blocks away. If we're supposed to be clocking ourselves on the hunger scale all the time, how exactly do we tell the difference between a reading of 4 and a reading of 6?'

'Everybody's different.' I told them, 'Basically, if you're not sure how hungry you are, the answer is Not Very.'

IF I'M NOT HUNGRY, WHAT AM I?

Ask yourself the question and figure out the answer

'Well,' Lisa said, 'I am definitely hungry, I could sit down and just eat plain bread right now without even thinking about that paté in the fridge. What are you making out of all this stuff anyway?'

'You get a choice. I'm doing tuna and chilli beans as well as chicken and broccoli. We'll have it with some brown rice and a salad.'

'I thought you were vegetarian?'

'I am, but that doesn't mean I can't cook meat sometimes. I eat fish anyway and there's no point in presenting people with an eating plan that's totally alien to them. Can you imagine Faye and Eve eating brown rice and Quorn every night?'

'I'm sure Faye needs chips to maintain that chest of hers,' said Mo. 'Can you imagine Faye flat chested? It would be like Marilyn Monroe's face on Twiggy's body. It would look like a transplant.' She picked up the paper and scanned the TV page. 'Why don't we eat on our laps, then we can watch AbFab.'

I started serving. 'Video it. I want you to enjoy this meal now, first time around, not eat it with half your mind on what Patsy and Eddie are doing. Try really concentrating on the food itself. Smell it first and decide which one you really want.'

'Pete, you're being weird on us again. Suppose we were in a restaurant. We can't really go around smelling everything, you're expected to read the menu, remember?'

'You don't have to have something under your nose to smell it. Just remember a few smells. If I say "bacon sandwich" to you, can you smell it? Even vegetarians, like me, can usually smell a bacon sandwich.'

The two of them were laughing and sniffing. Eventually Lisa took the tuna and Mo opted for the chicken.

'Don't forget,' I reminded them, 'you're not supposed to enjoy this.'

'Why not?'

'It's healthy.'

Dinner took a while. I was getting them to taste the food and tell me what they thought. Then we sat for a while and talked. 'Do you want anything else?' asked Lisa as she started to clear the table. 'We usually have some fruit or something, don't we Mo?'

'Well, I used to like something sweet to finish a meal. I've been programmed from birth to want something sweet when I've eaten my dinner. But since I'm on the diet too, it's always fruit now. Actually, I'm so full, I couldn't even eat a slice of Viennetta if we had one. Which we don't anymore. Do you remember that time we ate a whole one between us?'

'Don't remind me,' called Lisa from the kitchen. 'And it was mint which I don't even like.'

Would you rather waste food on your plate or on your waist?

'And we couldn't wait for it to get to room temperature, we were so desperate to get it down us.' Mo remembered. 'We were hacking away at it and it was so cold you couldn't taste it. So why am I feeling full right now when I haven't eaten as much as usual?'

'You just gave your body time to clock the food you put in it,' I said. 'And we talked about it and you thought about it while you were eating. You weren't thinking about anything else, you weren't watching television, or reading or working, were you? You were concentrating on the food itself.'

She nodded. 'Yes, I'm getting used to eating on its own and I'm definitely getting more pleasure out of what I eat.'

After dinner we washed up and I packed all the extra food into tubs for the following night. 'Let's take a walk down by the river.'

'It's late and I've got ironing to do,' Mo protested. 'You and Lisa go without me. We really took ages over dinner, didn't we?'

When we got out of the flat Lisa said, 'She's only staying in because she's hoping Chris will phone.'

'Sounds reasonable. Don't tell me you're jealous.'

'Of course not. It's ironic though, isn't it? Mo makes friends easier than me. She always has. She never sees the downside of anybody, or, if she does, she just overlooks it. It's the same with herself. Until she caught the dieting bug from me, she was pretty happy with herself and so were her boyfriends. And she was never short of a date. It wasn't till she met Chris that she started having doubts, if you know what I mean. Now, me, I've always been striving for perfection because I've always felt that when I'm perfect, I'll meet perfect people and have the perfect job.'

I turned to Lisa. 'What do you really want, right now?'

'Right now? A Galaxy caramel to round off that delicious dinner.' She looked longingly at BuyLate across the street.

'OK, I'll buy you one, if you can convince me that it's really what you want.'

'Of course it's what I want. They are just the closest thing to heaven.'

"Sad," I thought, but I actually said: 'What would a Galaxy caramel look like in your stomach?'

'Let me see, oh pretty disgusting.' She pulled a face.

'How would you feel an hour or half an hour after eating it?'

'Guilty, annoyed with myself, I'd have that sweet, sickly feeling in the back of my throat. You know, when you eat something you shouldn't have eaten, you can taste it forever.'

The greatest discovery of my generation is that a human being can alter his life by altering his attitudes of mind

William James

'Where would it go?'

'Straight on my hips. I don't need it right now.'

'What else could you eat that would feel better than the Galaxy caramel.'

'Oh, an apple, maybe. Or, no, really and truly I don't want anything to eat at all. It's a totally different feeling to the way I was just before we had dinner.'

'Maybe it's not hunger then. What else would satisfy the craving?'

She looked at me sideways and I felt a flicker of danger so I quickly added, 'What I mean is, maybe you need to sleep or walk or do a crossword or light some candles or stroke the cat or do some yoga or call your mother or...'

'I thought you were going to come up with something more interesting there. Never mind. I get your point. "Think Before You Eat", not "Eat Before You Think". Right?'

'Right.'

The following day, I finished my afternoon session in time to call on Lisa and collect the food which I'd left in her fridge overnight. She was working from home all day but there was too much for her to carry to the club. I rang the bell and looked down the steps through the basement window while I waited. I could see her workstation on the table. I could also see a couple of plates, a cereal bowl and what looked like a Ryvita pack. I guessed she probably wouldn't be feeling great when she answered the door.

'Thank goodness you're here. I hate working from home,' she said as I followed her down to the kitchen.

'Why? Don't you get a lot done?'

'Yes, but I miss the company. Then, when I'm actually at work I want peace and quiet to concentrate. I know, I'm impossible.'

'I don't think I've ever heard you say anything nice about yourself Lisa. Don't you ever give yourself credit for doing something right?'

'Credit for what? Eating as many Hobnobs as I've typed paragraphs?'

'All I could see through the window was a Ryvita wrapper.'

'You're spying on me. OK, I know if you eat enough Ryvita they turn to fat just like Hobnobs. What the hell. I don't care any more.'

'Yes you do. It doesn't matter how few biscuits you've eaten or how many paragraphs you've typed or whether you're a size 8 or a size 12. You're permanently dissatisfied with your own performance at everything, slimming, working, exercising.'

You've got to create a dream. You've got to uphold the dream.

Eric Burdon

'Yes, what else?'

'Nothing. But listen to me now. Suppose I were to ask you, seriously, what you really want, what would you say?'

'Is this one of those exercises you gave us? The What-Do-You-Want parts 1 to 69? I'm not doing too well with those.'

'Why don't you do it with Mo?'

'She's got Chris.'

'Alright then, do it with me. What do you want?'

'I want to get rid of all this lard I'm carrying round on my butt.'

'You cannot be more than a couple of pounds outside your ideal weight.'

'Six and a half pounds. Exactly.'

'And for six and a half pounds you spend every waking moment thinking about dieting and deprivation? Anyway, answer the question. What do you want?'

'If you buy six pounds of lard at Tesco, it takes up quite a bit of space in the trolley. I want to lose that six and a half pounds and keep it lost.'

'What pictures do you see when you say that to yourself?'

'I picture myself with thirteen or fourteen packs of lard moulded on to me from the waist down and I think, "if I could just scrape that off and start from scratch." But it doesn't work like that.'

'Suppose you were to say "I want to be slim and fit".'

'What's the difference?'

'What do you see when you turn it around like that?'

'I can't see pictures, if that's what you mean. Funny really, because I always thought the madder you were, the more likely you would be to see things that weren't there!'

Whatever she said, I could tell she was actually making pictures in her mind by the way she was looking up all the time at an imaginary screen above her head. 'Alright, I know you can't visualise things very clearly. Just try a couple of easy ones for me. Picture your front door.'

Lisa looked up at a point on curtain rail. 'Yes, of course, I can picture the door, that's different.'

'Now try a harder one. What do you see in that same spot on the curtain rail when you say to yourself, "I want to be slim and fit"?'

Don't bury your feelings under food

'I see me, on a beach, in a bikini. I'm running into the sea, laughing. You know, just like one of those travel ads you get on TV just after Christmas when you're at your fattest and most depressed.'

'Is it nice and clear and bright?'

'No, it's just a fuzzy little impression I have.'

I reached up towards the curtain rail and brought my hand down to a foot in front of her face. 'If I bring it right up close, what difference does that make?'

She was looking intently at my hand. 'It's much closer and clearer, like looking at a holiday photo.'

'In colour?'

'Oh, yes.' Lisa's cheeks were pink, suddenly. And she hadn't even put her make-up on, I noticed.

'How does that make you feel, seeing yourself looking great in a bikini?'

'Well, great, of course.'

'And how does the other picture make you feel, the one with you trying to scrape the lard off your butt?'

'Depressed, hopeless, hungry.'

'Hungry?'

'When everything looks hopeless, it's time to eat. You've got nothing else to lose. And don't start on about feelings because I've been writing them all down in my diary. I knew all of that already.'

'Knew what?'

'I eat when I feel like a failure and when I'm lonely, or nervous.'

'That's because you're focusing on being lonely and nervous. Your mind is like a heat-seeking missile. What you point it at is what you get. It's a good idea to point it at something you want, like being slim, happy, successful or whatever. Do you think that if you were to picture yourself every day, looking great, running along that beach, you'd still be stuffing yourself with comfort food? Of course you wouldn't, because that behaviour wouldn't fit with your self image.'

Lisa looked doubtful.

'OK,' I said, 'if I can't convince you about the positive potential you have, let's get back to the problems. Let's think of a "for instance". Why were you nervous before Mo's party?'

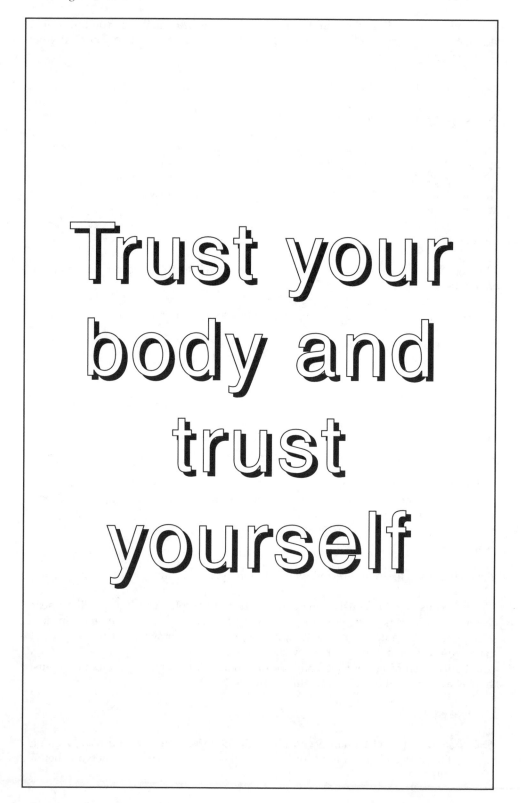

Trust your body and trust yourself

She looked at me angrily. 'Give me a break will you? Everybody has their eating triggers. Those are mine. Now, Mo, she eats when she's depressed. Didn't you notice how unhappy she was at her birthday?'

'Well of course I did, but why? Mo used to love parties. Any party. Anybody's party.'

Lisa shook her head. 'That was BC. She wanted to actually be at the party with him but he wouldn't. He didn't have to go to that in drag. Not in my opinion. I don't know what he's playing at but it's not good for Mo.'

'OK, don't distract me Lisa, what do you want?'

She paused at the fridge door and turned to face me. 'I want to be slim of course, what the hell do you think I want? How long have you known me?'

'Well, if you know that's what you want, why do you keep telling yourself what you don't want? You say you want to lose weight. Well, why the hell aren't you focusing on being slim? Why do you keep looking at yourself covered in lard?'

'Alright. Let's play the game. I want to be slim.'

'How will you know when you're as slim as you want to be?'

'I suppose I'll be happy.'

'It sounds to me that you're looking for an answer to the meaning of life and we all know that's forty two. What else in your life will improve when you're as slim as you want to be?'

'I'll feel confident.' She sounded more thoughtful now.

'Can you think of some resources you have got which can help you achieve what you want?'

'What are you on Pete? Sometimes you are completely out of touch.'

'Humour me. Answer the question. I cooked you dinner last night. You owe me.'

'Stop snapping your fingers at me will you? I hate it when you do that. OK. I'm determined. I have a lot of determination. I don't give up easily.'

'Wait a minute, what about all the diets you've given up on?'

'Maybe, but I always started another one. I'm never not on a diet. Diets are like men. It's nice to have a change once in a while.'

'Instead of relying on a diet, why not rely on yourself for a change?'

She was stacking up the food containers in a carrier bag. 'Are you suggesting I should give up men or dieting?'

'Just dieting.'

Lisa handed me the carrier bags with a strange smile. 'That's a relief.'

Chapter Six

Cakes And Sweet Desserts

As I loaded the back of the car I tried to remember when Lisa last had a regular boyfriend. But by the time I'd struggled through the rush hour traffic I wasn't thinking about anything but getting organised for the group. I'd printed out a stack of posters which I stuck all the way up from the entrance to the top of the stairs:

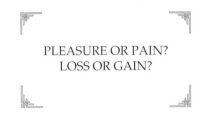

PLEASURE OR PAIN?
LOSS OR GAIN?

was all they said, plus the time and room and "Pete Cohen's Lighten Up Sessions" on the bottom. I was bringing some plates and forks and spoons up from the kitchen when I met Miriam coming down.

'Hello, I just popped up to see how you're getting on. Looks like you're having a party tonight. What happened? You think they might have taken too many Fat Burning Pills last week?'

'It's alright Miriam. It's going to be delicious, nutritious and slimming.'

'Nonsense, all food is fattening.'

'No, all food is fuel, you just have to burn the right amount. Anyway, we're all going to the Duke's Head later, so I have to make sure they've left room for the pork scratchings. Why don't you join us?'

'How sweet of you. I might.'

As she clicked back down the stairs on her spiky heels she passed the rest of the group coming up. Mo and Lisa trailed behind chatting to Ben and Lewis. I looked for Chris. I'd been wondering what gender he'd turn up in, but he didn't seem to be around.

'As you know, we're finishing this evening with something to eat. I hope the fitness freaks got the message about the aerobics being cancelled for tonight. Now, how about your food diaries for last week?'

I'm at the age where I think more about food than sex

Last week I put a mirror over my dining room table

Rodney Dangerfield

'Here we go,' said Lewis. 'Bloody feelings again. I'll have you know Pete that, thanks to you, we didn't even get a pizza in with the game last Wednesday. Ben wouldn't have it. We'll be sitting around drinking camomile tea and doing male bonding soon. If you don't get this weight off me in the next five weeks mate, I'm out of here.'

Faye and Eve had managed to seat themselves between Ben and Lewis, deliberately I suspected. 'Did you say bondage, Sweetheart?' Faye enquired innocently. Is that something to do with the pain and pleasure?'

'We don't need to talk about your feelings,' I said quickly. 'The aim of the diary is to help you know yourselves better, not to expose you to the rest of the world, or even the group. Once you're aware of your own eating and exercise patterns you can make changes. And I mean little, specific, changes. Just change one, or at most, two, things at a time. Diets that insist you change your whole life in one go are unlikely to work. Be gentler with yourself than that. If you know there are dangerous times of day for you, or dangerous emotions or dangerous activities, you can see what a big difference a little change can make. Let's ask Ben, for example, if he enjoyed the match any the less because of the lack of the pizza?'

He shook his head. 'Not really.'

'Well I did,' said Lewis.

'I never could pay any mind to the pizza if it was a good game,' Ben added. 'And the problem this week was Lewis whining about his pizza all the way through the game so nobody else could concentrate.'

Faye was dying to tell us something so I nodded at her. 'I actually cooked Sunday lunch for my son and his father,' she said. 'We don't eat together that often. Anyway, the two of them went to the pub and didn't get back till half past three. It was all dried up. I just binned it and went for a walk.'

'I'd have tipped it over them when they did get in,' remarked Eve.

'Well,' continued Faye, 'by the evening, I was in on my own and I suddenly realised I was hungry. I mean, 9 ¾ on the hunger scale, I'd missed lunch and I didn't have time for breakfast, so, you know what I did?'

Lewis sighed, loudly.

'I'd made a lemon meringue, it's Sean's favourite. It was still in the fridge, so I just ate the lot. There was some ice cream as well so I had that with it.'

'Ice cream and lemon meringue, surely not,' came a voice from the back row.

Lisa spoke for the first time. 'Coffee ice cream and lemon meringue. Yummy.'

'Why didn't you have a sandwich or something first and then just take a slice of the pudding?' I asked Faye.

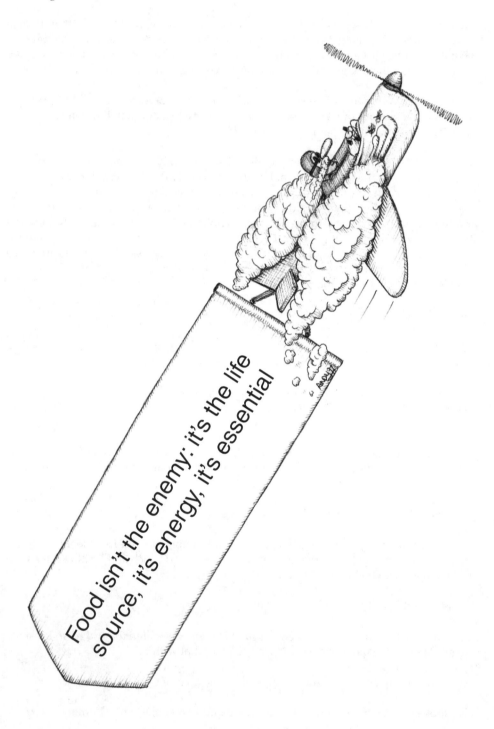

Food isn't the enemy: it's the life source, it's energy, it's essential

'I couldn't be bothered. Too much effort. I was making a point. It wasn't my fault, it was their fault for not being there. I was lonely and depressed and ugly and nobody loved me. All of those reasons.'

I could have wept for her and I could see that a few other people felt the same. Lisa and Mo were at the back, perched on their chairs like a couple of miserable London pigeons, one plump and gloomy, one thin and fluttery. 'Faye, that sounds like a real bummer of a Sunday. The odds were stacked against you. It sounds like you had all your difficult pattern buttons pressed at the same time. Other people, your own feelings, time of day, all of that.'

Eve patted her shoulder. 'I think you did bloody well to stop at the pudding and ice cream. I'd probably have eaten my way through anything else that came to hand once I'd started.'

'I might have done,' agreed Faye, 'but I didn't have much in. Now there's just me and Sean most of the time, I don't bother. He isn't usually in for meals. I did put my coat on though and I was on my way to BuyLate when I thought to myself, "ten minute walk, there and back. If I add on an extra bit I can get as far as Eve's house." So I didn't stop at the shop. I just went for a walk and stuck my 5p in the jar when I got home.'

'I thought you called in for your catalogue.'

'That was just an excuse.'

'Well done,' I told her. 'One of the things I want you all to start doing for the next week is to catch yourselves doing something right and give yourselves some credit for it. That's definitely a situation when Faye should have literally given herself a pat on the back.'

'What, for eating a lemon meringue pie and the best part of a tub of cookie dough ice cream?'

'No, for not eating anything else after that, despite extreme provocation, and for taking a walk instead. Just think how you'd have responded to the same situation a few weeks ago. Everybody who's a success has done it by mastering failure, and that's exactly what you did.'

'Oh, yes, even a couple of weeks ago, I'd have bought the biscuits. No question. But you know, by the time I got home again, the craving was gone. I read that on a calendar and it's true. "Cravings are like waves, they reach a peak and then they die away".'

'You mean there's a calendar for slimmers?' enquired Lewis. 'What are the pictures of? Fat people to frighten you or thin ones to inspire you?'

'No pictures, just quotes and recipes,' Faye replied. 'My husband gave it to me before we split up.' Then she added quietly, 'Bastard.'

AN EATING PLAN

Only you can know *exactly* what and when you need to eat. But everybody needs a variety of foods from different foods groups. This will help you to get the energy, protein, vitamins, minerals, and fibre you need for good health.

I split the groups into eight:

Vegetables
Fruits
Cereals, grains and bread
Beans and lentils
Meat, fish, poultry, soya or tofu
Dairy products
Fats
Sugar

'Well,' I said, 'I think that Faye should give herself some credit. A lot of people spend time feeling bad about themselves. They plan for it because they expect to feel bad. How about planning to have some fun and feeling good instead? It's a matter of where you put your attention. If you spend a lot of time practising feeling bad, so it won't upset you when it happens, it can get to be a habit. Focus on the good bits more often. When you get something right, congratulate yourself. Do it every day, there's always some little thing you've got right, even if it's not eating a biscuit or walking to the bus. I mean literally. Pat yourselves on the back.' I wondered if this would be physically possible for Faye so I turned towards her and started clapping. Everybody else joined in. She was lost for words.

And I figured it was time to get onto the less emotional subject of exercise.

How do you feel about exercise?
Would you like to do more?
What's stopping you?

I'd written it up on the flip chart and answers were coming in thick and fast.

'Because it's not fun,' suggested Lisa. 'You know me, I've tried loads of times. I come to the gym, then I give up again. I even bought one of those rowing machines…'

'I know, I fall over it every time I try to walk down your hallway. When did you last use it?'

'For about three weeks before I went to Greece last summer. I'm going to sell it if anybody's interested.' She looked around the room and smiled. 'It's great for sporting injuries.'

'You mean you can use it for building up your strength when you're recovering from a fall or something?' asked Ben, looking interested.

'No, I'm talking about causing injuries. It wasn't just Pete who tripped over it. My mum was standing on it to dust the pictures in the hall last time she came to visit, but she slipped off and sprained her ankle. She said it proved keeping fit was dangerous.'

'When I was at school,' said Faye, 'I was always the last to be picked for a team when everybody had to play netball. I left at 16 and I swear it wasn't because of the exams, it was because I couldn't face another winter freezing to death on the hockey pitch.'

'I don't remember exercising at school,' said Lisa. 'I realised early on it was either going to be life-threatening or humiliating or both. I used to be in the loo fixing my mascara so I could make a fast getaway later.'

Lewis had been shaking his head in disbelief for some time. 'Excuse me for disagreeing with all this expertise and experience, but for me the sport was the best part of being at school.'

PRINCIPLES OF A HEALTHY DIET

Maintaining a healthy weight

Choosing a diet low in fat, saturated fat and cholesterol

Eating plenty of fruit, vegetables and grain products which provide essential energy, vitamins, minerals, fibre and complex carbohydrates. They are low in dietary fat and help to lower your intake of fat

Using sugars in moderation because the body easily converts them to fat and they don't provide the nutrients your body needs

Minimising use of salt can help reduce the risk of high blood pressure

Ben agreed. 'They were glory days. I was in the first team. But, you know, it's very hard to carry on at that level. Unless you're good enough to take it up professionally, you get locked into a job that involves sitting down all day. I even gave up working out because I couldn't do it the way I used to. And because I wouldn't compromise I lost it completely. Since I've realised that these strict diets aren't really for me, I've decided to go for the exercise option and just eat sensibly. I'm walking and I've started jogging again. The trouble is, I'm not really enjoying it. There doesn't seem to be much point when you're not working towards something, training for something, does there? It was partly being in a team and competing that kept me motivated.'

'Personally,' said Eve, 'I think when you get older, you just see exercise as a necessary evil, don't you? I'd rather get in the car any day than even walk to the bus stop and I think we all feel like that if we're honest. If it wasn't meant to hurt you wouldn't have Jane Fonda going on about "no pain, no gain", would you? Quite honestly, I don't have time to get into one of those bloody daft outfits and take myself off to classes every evening. Apart from the fact that the work would be stacking up at home, it's embarrassing and I don't enjoy it.'

'But Eve,' I moved towards her, 'you've been walking more, you told me. That's pretty good exercise. This theory that it's got to hurt is nonsense and it's the reason why so many people start and don't continue. If you push yourself to exhaustion and you're bored rigid, of course you're going to give up. You'd be daft not to. Let's get back to pleasure and pain. I'm going to prove to you that you can all, every one of you, do some regular exercise and it won't hurt, it won't bore you, you're going to love it.'

'Eventually,' muttered Mo at the back.

'Eventually, or even sooner than that. But I'm not promising you a quick fix.'

'What about resistance training?' asked Lewis.

'I suppose you mean resistance to training.' There was no escape from Faye's sense of humour now she'd got her weekend's trauma off her impressive chest.

'Why don't you come right up here and explain the benefits of resistance training, Lewis?'

He didn't get up. 'It just means that you get more benefit from exercise if you're working against some resistance. Like walking, the road is your resistance, with cycling, it's the gears and so on.'

'Lewis is right,' I told them. 'It's no big deal. It's just that the main benefit of exercise from a weight loss point of view is to tone your muscles and make them leaner so they burn fat more efficiently. If you're working against resistance, you're working them harder. Muscles have special enzymes that enable them to burn up tremendous amounts of calories in a short period. The more well-toned muscles you have, the more calories they need to maintain their function. You want to metabolise more fat? Muscles account for 90% of your metabolism, so if you're eating 1,500 calories, 1,350 will be burned in the muscles.

HOW MUCH OF WHAT YOU FANCY?

How much you eat depends on how much your body needs. The only way to know this is to get to know yourself and that's where the Hunger Scale can help.

A lot of people like the fact that diets tell them when and what to eat. But that's not what this is about. The Food Cake is a guide to what types of food you should be eating but only you will know how much. And you do it by listening to your body so you can eat when you're hungry and stop when you're full.

What's more, that special enzyme which only exists in your muscles can increase calorie burning fifty fold during exercise. If you want to burn calories, then look to the quality and quantity of your muscles. If you lose muscle, your need for calories diminishes and you turn more calories into fat. The more toned muscle you have, the more calories those muscles need and the quicker your metabolism works.'

'OK, you've convinced me. I want more muscles,' said Faye. 'Do I have to use my own or can I just get the benefit from somebody else's. Sylvester Stallone, maybe? Sorry Lewis, Sorry,' she caught his expression. 'I tell you what, I'll ask a sensible question.'

'Hooray,' muttered Lewis.

Faye continued. 'I'm walking regularly, I'm running up my stairs. And, I admit, I can see a difference and feel a difference, even if the scales can't. But what I want to know is how I know when I'm doing it right or when I'm doing enough? And don't start banging on about getting to know yourself and personal blueprints. I wouldn't generate my own chemicals any more than I'd make my own wine. You're looking at a woman who's so out of touch with herself she can eat a whole lemon meringue.'

Ben put his hand on her shoulder. 'Faye, you will know when you've got it right. But what you need to do is start gradually. Whether you're walking, or swimming, or dancing, or whatever it is you do, just start slowly and build up to the level when you're breathless but you're still feeling comfortable. Maintain your pace for fifteen minutes. Like Pete says, "keep whistling and talking".'

'I can't whistle,' said Faye.

'Never mind,' said Eve. 'Let's stick to the talking. We can do that.'

'Don't we know it,' said Lewis.

I started to set out the food I'd brought with me and invited them to try it.

'Is this the sort of thing that we're meant to be eating at home?' asked Eve. 'My family would never eat this. I'm not sure about it myself.'

'It's great,' Mo told her. 'Pete cooked this for us last night and you can take my word for it. Cooking's my business and I'm definitely going to use these recipes.'

'I shouldn't think you could serve food like this commercially and charge for it, could you?' asked Lewis, 'After all, it's the sort of thing people eat in squats, isn't it?'

That was the time I came closest to physical violence. But while I was taking some deep breaths to restrain myself, Eve weighed back in.

'I take back what I said. It's really nice. It tastes more like real food than I expected. The problem is, Pete, if you work like I do, and you've got teenagers to feed, it's actually quite difficult to cook every night. I like those ready-meals or we have takeaways. I'm not Wonder Woman, I can't do everything.'

HAVE YOUR CAKE AND EAT IT

The food cake is an eating plan that works on the principle that you need to eat a variety of foods from the eight different food groups I've defined.

Example Of The Daily Food Cake

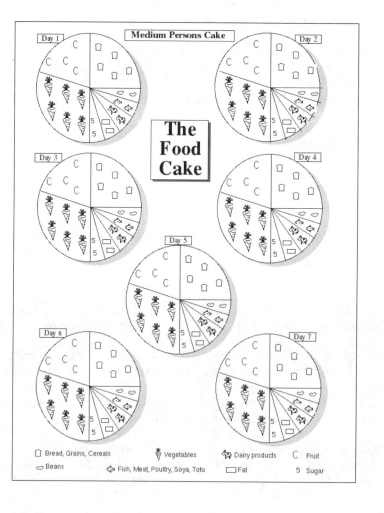

'Recipes like this don't actually take that long to prepare. And you'll be doing yourself such a favour if you take that little extra bit of time. Plus you'll save a lot of money. Those pre-prepared meals are expensive and if you go for the diet options they cost even more.' While I was talking I noticed that Lewis was helping himself to more of the chicken and broccoli.

'So, is this what you call a healthy diet?' called somebody from the back.

'Yes, it's a good balance of carbohydrate, protein and fibre with a lot of fresh veggies and no processed food. It's also very low in fat. We'll be talking about healthy diets in more detail later on. The reason I'm feeding you tonight is because it's pleasure and pain week and I'm trying to make the point that healthy food can be pleasurable. Does anybody dare to disagree with me?'

'It was alright,' said Lewis. 'We were planning to go for a kebab later anyway.'

'OK, let's round it up for tonight. Remember, pleasure and pain. The biggest factor you have to contend with is thinking that taking action will be more painful than not taking any action at all. It's not true. Just take the steps you feel you can take towards exercise and a healthy diet one at a time.

You're going to start making some different links in your mind and break some old ones. Pain can be your friend if you unhook it from healthy eating and lots of exercise. Start putting some pain into the effect that all that inactivity is having on your body. Exercise in a way that gives you pleasure, try some food that's good for you and tastes delicious too. Let's put it another way. You're re-programming your brain. One line of code at a time. That should appeal to you Lewis.'

It seemed like most of the class had decided to go to the Duke's Head. Maybe they just wanted to wash down the tuna and chilli bean supper. Ben and Lewis may have had other motives. "May the best man win," I thought, as I watched them follow Lisa down the stairs. We'd just settled in the Duke's Head when I nearly fell off my seat. Miriam was walking towards us carrying what I suspected was a glass of mineral water. She smiled at everybody, 'I thought I'd take you up on your invitation.'

It was obvious she knew quite a few of the group and several people greeted her, some with warmth and some with embarrassment. Then there was an awkward silence.

'Well,' she said, brightly, 'what have you been discovering this evening?'

'We've been talking about muscles and we've just had an interesting meal,' Eve told her.

'So you have been eating at your diet class?' Miriam raised her eyebrows. 'What an original approach.'

You may not be sure whether you're a small, medium or large person, but don't worry about it. You'll soon have a much better idea of how much you really need to eat when you're taking a little more exercise and tuning in to your body's needs.

I suggest that everybody stays with two servings each of protein, dairy products, fat and sugar, regardless of size. If you need to eat more, then increase your vegetables, fruit and carbohydrates – not your lard, cream or red meat!

I made a space for her to sit down beside me and then I turned back to Eve. 'Talking about muscles, Eve, one other thing you need to remember,' I said, 'you can't build muscle overnight and you probably won't see a weight loss to begin with. What will happen is that you will start to look and feel slimmer because muscle is heavier than the fat it's replacing.'

'Muscle weighs more than fat! Isn't that a bit of an old chestnut?' Miriam asked. 'We'd all like to believe it of course,' she added.

'Oh, I believe it,' said Faye. 'See this skirt?'

She stood up and we were all transfixed. I prayed she wasn't going to hitch her sweater up too high. It was years since I'd been thrown out of a pub. She turned around and discreetly tucked two fingers into her waistband. 'I couldn't do that a couple of weeks ago, but the scales don't show that much difference.' She sat down again and smacked Lewis in the stomach. 'If you do what Pete tells you, you'll be able to do that again soon, maybe you'll even be able to stop wearing those ridiculous braces. Honestly, Mickey Mouse at your age!'

Lewis was visibly irritated and slightly winded. He obviously fancied himself as rather a cool dresser but the result was Used Car Salesman rather than City Trader. Still, as Faye said last week, it was probably better than looking like a programmer. Once again Ben had upstaged him and was looking pretty cool in black and white. He looked like a domino.

I intervened. 'You and Ben have been super-fit in the past. The problem is that when you stop exercising you sometimes carry on eating, and men have a tendency to store their excess fat round the middle.'

'Now there's a polite way of saying Lewis has a beer belly.' Eve seemed determined to stir things up.

Ben was determined to lower the temperature. 'If you've been fit and you let yourself get out of shape, it is much harder to find a compromise. Lewis and I have to recognise that we are effectively starting from scratch. Just like the rest of you.'

'Like the rest of us weaklings and fatties you mean?' Lisa suggested. But she was smiling at him, for the first time this evening.

Ben smiled at her and continued. 'I can tell you all from my own first hand experience that exercise feels good when you do it regularly. You get a high from the endorphins you generate that, as far as I can remember, beats any drug (legal of course) that I've ever taken. The problem me and Lewis have got is that we're never going to be in the kind of condition we were ten years ago. Our lives have changed, we can't spend all our time working out and eating out while somebody pays the bills. I think we both have to find a more balanced way and I can tell you, it's been difficult for me to know what I really want to do.' He was looking at Lisa and I wondered what he was talking about.

WHAT'S A SERVING?

If you want to see if you are getting enough fruit, vegetables and carbohydrates, one serving is a small tea or coffee cup or American measuring cup filled flat, not heaped.

Fruit	1 large fruit (apple, orange, peach) ¼ cup of fresh juice 1 cup of berries or pineapple 20 cherries or 20 grapes
Cereals, Grains and Bread	1 cup of cooked rice, pasta, potatoes 1 cup of unsweetened cereal 2 slices of bread or 2 small rolls
Meat, Poultry, Fish, Soya, Tofu	3oz lean meat, poultry, fish, soya or tofu
Vegetables, beans or lentils	1 cup of cooked vegetables
Dairy Foods	1 egg 2oz low fat cheese 1 cup non fat milk ½ cup semi-skimmed milk ½ cup low fat yoghurt
Fat	1 tablespoon of oil, margarine, butter 4 tablespoons of cream 12 mixed nuts 40 unsalted peanuts 20 almonds 4 teaspoons of peanut butter 30 crisps, 16 chips, 2 biscuits
Sugar	1 tablespoon of sugar, honey or jam

'I think you've done brilliantly.' Lisa was simpering at him. 'I wish I could shed a few pounds just where I wanted to.'

'Well you can't,' Faye told her. 'Women always lose weight from the places they least want to lose weight from. Isn't that true, Pete?'

'I'm afraid so. Women were designed to store their emergency fat layer on their bums and thighs. If they start to shed it that's the last place it leaves from. Same with men and the beer belly.'

'So much for spot reduction then.' Mo was thinking aloud. 'I tried it once. I worked on my thigh muscles for weeks so I wouldn't look flabby in shorts and by the time I finished I had legs like tree trunks. I didn't look flabby though. More like a Russian shot putter.'

'Nothing, short of surgery, will give you spot reduction. You were increasing your muscle mass but not reducing the fat,' I told her. 'Fat isn't attached to any particular muscle. However many sit-ups and leg-lifts you did you were only building up the muscles involved. Most women will lose weight from the top down which is usually the opposite of what they want.'

'We women were never designed to look like men. We don't have completely flat stomachs but we are meant to have thighs, hips and bums,' said Eve. 'It's just that mine are a bit out of control.'

'Well,' said Miriam, 'you have had a busy evening learning all about your body chemistry and physiology by the sound of it. The question I have for you, girls and boys' (I cringed), 'the question I have is, have you lost any weight?'

I had to field that one. 'Actually, Miriam, when you lose something, like your car keys for example, you usually end up finding it again, don't you? No-one in the Lighten Up group has lost anything, they're working towards finding a better body size and shape for the future.'

'That's right, Love,' said Eve, 'I've gained two pounds of slimness.' Everybody laughed.

Miriam waved her hands at us dismissively. 'I'm afraid I'm rather confused.'

I was confused too, but I assumed Eve was trying to be helpful. 'Miriam, listen to me. The real issue is not the weight. Weight is the symptom of the problem. If it was the whole problem, all you would have to do is lose weight successfully one time and the problem would be solved. The real problem is whatever causes the over-eating. If you resolve this, then the problem will be solved.'

'Sounds a bit psychological to me.'

'I'm not talking about digging around in people's psyches. All I mean is that over-eating is caused by learned eating behaviour, it's emotional eating. You need to trust your body, listen to your body, trust your feelings and accept yourself. We were born with bodies that knew how to eat perfectly and we were taught to ignore that

We were born with bodies
that only wanted food
when we needed it

Overeating and eating
when we are not hungry
has been caused by
learned eating habits

*All you need to do is
re-discover your
natural relationship
with food*

knowledge. You know the statistics as well as I do, Miriam. 75-80% of US women diet and hate their bodies. Hating your body causes you to overeat from shame, self disgust and despair.'

'I know, Dear, that's where I come in. Fatness is caused by too much food. It's as simple as that. I give my clients a diet that gets them back to the body shape they want and then they can be happy with themselves again.'

'It's the wrong way round. Dieting and controlling food doesn't help because most people learned to eat as a mechanism for coping with their feelings. You're prescribing the problem to solve the problem. Unless you can cope with your feelings some other way and recover your natural relationship with food and eating you will never stay slim.'

'Well, of course you don't stay slim unless you keep up your diet. Really Peter, you're reinventing the wheel, only you're making it square. Anyway, it's been very interesting but I must dash. Enjoy your evening.'

Mo left soon after Miriam but Lisa seemed to be enjoying herself for once and hardly acknowledged her leaving. The group didn't break up until last orders and I saw Lewis lean over to Lisa and whisper something in her ear. She shook her head and smiled.

Ben, was sitting across the table from her. He obviously made a guess at what Lewis had said. 'I don't have my car here, Lisa, but I can walk you home.'

She looked uncertain for a minute and I stood up and touched her shoulder. 'I'll give you a lift, it's not often I bring the car so I might as well justify it.'

Both Lewis and Ben gave me withering looks. Lewis shrugged his shoulders. 'Coming Ben? We could call in for a game of pool on the way back.'

'I thought you were going for a kebab.'

'I was only winding Pete up. To be honest, I'm still full after those bloody lentils he fed us. I'll say one thing for beans, they soak up the beer.'

'And give you energy?' I suggested.

'For what?'

Lisa didn't invite me in, and I noticed the lights were on in the downstairs flat as she got out of the car. I didn't see any of them around the following week and I was wondering if the next Friday's Lighten Up class was going to be as lively as the last one.

When Friday came around, to my amazement, Chris was there, wearing jeans and no makeup. I saw Lewis and Ben glance at him and say something to each other as they came in.

'Well, boys and girls,' I began...

Never give in. Never, never, never, never.

Winston Churchill

'Who says men aren't bitchy,' Faye interrupted. 'Leave Miriam alone, Pete, she's doing her best.'

'Unworthy,' commented Chris, raising elegant eyebrows at me. His eyebrows were the only give-away when he was having a male day.

I felt a bit ashamed of myself so I launched into the food cake. It's always a winner. 'You'll like this,' I told them. 'It's an eating plan, sort of.'

When I'd explained it and sketched it all out on the flip chart Eve said, 'That's more like it, you know where you are with something like that, don't you? Why the heck didn't you give us that at the beginning?'

'Because I didn't want you to start relying on lists again. I wanted you to start listening to yourselves, learning what your own bodies needed and using the hunger scale. This is just a way of showing you how balanced your diet is because each time you have a particular food you just colour it in.'

'Painting by numbers,' muttered Lewis.

'Well, I agree, it's not rocket science, but that's the whole point. Some of the diet books in the American Top Ten need a nutritionist to work them out and a personal trainer on hand to tell you what to eat and how and when to exercise. What I'm giving you is the kind of stuff that your sub-conscious will learn and get on with while you go out and get a life.' I spotted the unrest before it happened and added hastily, 'Not that you haven't all got lives already.'

Eve waved her food cake information to get my attention. 'I'm beginning to like the idea of only eating when I'm hungry and eating what I want. I can see this is different from the normal diet sheet because it's telling you what foods you really ought to be eating rather than what you shouldn't. Am I right, Pete?'

'Yes, that's the idea. If you had a high performance sports car, what type of petrol and oil would you put in? How often would you clean it and check it over? You wouldn't put the wrong fuel in, would you? You wouldn't miss a service, would you?'

'I used to have a high performance body,' said Lewis unexpectedly.

Eve was sitting behind him and she leaned forwards, putting her hands on his shoulders. 'Don't worry, Love, looks aren't everything. At least, that's what my husband tells me.'

Faye wasn't going to miss this one. 'I'm sure you've still got what it takes,' she added, patting his arm.

I waited for the explosion. Nothing happened. Then Lewis said, 'the only high performance vehicle I've got now is the BMW. You can't be the person you were in your twenties.'

YOU ARE
WHAT YOU EAT

Think of your body as a high
performance sports car.

You would put the best quality
petrol and oil into it wouldn't you?

How about putting the right fuel
into your body?... fuel that allows
you to become slimmer, fitter and
healthier.

It's just a thought

Suddenly, Lisa stood up and screamed at him. 'That is total crap, Lewis. Why don't you pull yourself together. You can look and feel as good as you want to. You just don't want to make the effort.'

That did the trick. Lewis spun round on his seat. 'Alright, Miss Bloody Perfection,' he said, 'at least I'm realistic. If I looked like a damned stick insect wearing Prada you wouldn't find me wasting my time on a Friday night at a diet class.'

Just when you think you're in for a relatively straightforward evening when you're going to give everybody what they want and they're going to be grateful for it, it all goes pear shaped. I've noticed it before.

'Shh, both of you. Let's get back to the food cake.' I was watching Lisa out of the corner of my eye. Thankfully she wasn't crying. She looked more shocked than upset. 'What you put into your body not only affects what you look like, it also affects how well your body works, how you feel, your energy levels and your state of health.'

Mo put her hand up. 'Sometimes I want to feel like Banoffee Pie – all smooth and sticky'.

'If Ben was a pudding he'd definitely be Death By Chocolate,' said Lisa, completely out of the blue.

There was a stunned silence. I battled on.

It was a relief when the hour was over and the room emptied. I hoped nobody was going to want to stay behind and chat. But, as I was stacking the chairs, I heard the door open behind me. It was Lewis. 'I forgot my bag,' he said, picking it up from under his seat.

'What's that for? It looks heavy.'

'I've got to go in to the office and do some emergency work tonight so I thought I'd take something with me to eat. Since you got us going on this Hunger Scale I've started listening to my stomach and the canteen closes in the evening.'

'So you take something with you? Good idea. If you physically need to eat, then eat.'

'Not easy though, is it? I was brought up to eat at mealtimes and then I just added the snacks in between and that was it. I never gave myself a long enough gap to feel hungry as such.'

'And what's it like now you are?'

'Now I'm letting myself feel hungry? It still doesn't feel right. But once you know what it is, it's pretty good. Like an itch. And you have to scratch. By the way, who was the new guy tonight? He looked familiar, but I just couldn't place him. Neither could Ben.'

If you're going to do something wrong, at least enjoy doing it

Leo Roster

'Oh, nobody you'd know.' I didn't find Lewis easy to relate to, but I knew he hadn't come back just to try and find out who Chris was. I felt some responsibility so I asked the question. 'Do you really think you'll never get back into shape again?'

'I look like an ex-rugby player going to seed. I used to look like a Greek God.'

'What? Come in please?'

He grinned at me for the first time, ever, I think. 'There was a report on the back page of the local paper about ten years ago on a big club game when I was just about at my fittest. It was a standing joke at the time: "the game was saved by Lewis Jones, our local Greek God".'

'The reporter wasn't a woman by any chance, was she?' I asked.

'How did you guess? Of course, it got pinned up on the club Board and I thought I'd never hear the end of it. But I kind of liked it. In a way. No shortage of talent that year.'

'Most people put on weight as they get older, Lewis. It's just that for sportspeople like you, the change is more dramatic. But you can reverse the process. I can't promise you'll be a Greek God again. I believe you have to be around twenty to qualify. But you can look and feel good, in fact better than you did then. Remember all the injuries and hangovers? Do you really want to go through all that again? Just because you're past thirty doesn't mean you're past looking good. Think about the men women fall for. Robert Redford must qualify for a bus pass and Al Pacino is no spring chicken.'

I nearly added, 'you don't have to look like a slob,' but I decided that, even with our new rapport, it would be taking a risk. Lewis was still too big and aggressive looking to randomly annoy.

'Well, you'll be pleased to know that the Fat Jar is filling up on my mantelpiece,' he said. 'I don't have too much problem with getting a bit more exercise into the routine, it's just that I really don't think I can cope with counting up how many lentils I've eaten every day, much less colouring them in. Do me a favour Pete, I may not always act like it, but I am a grown-up now.'

'You don't have to do anything weird with your lifestyle to make the changes you want to make. You can reverse the process, mostly by adding some more activity to your schedule and with just a little bit of change to your eating habits. For example,' I reached over and grabbed the can of cola sticking out of his bag. 'do you have any idea of how many spoonfuls of sugar there are in here?'

'No.'

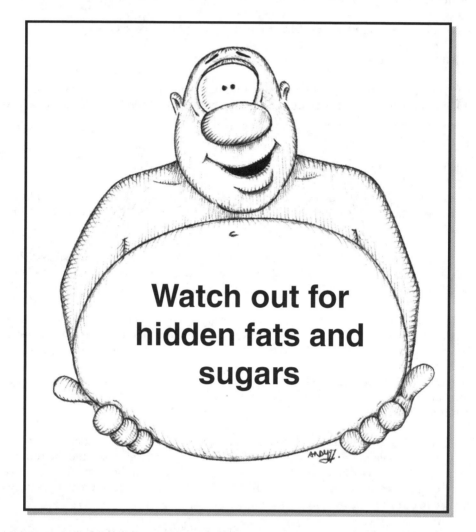

Did you know that most soft drinks
have the equivalent
of fifteen teaspoons of sugar
in them?

'Fifteen. So if you cut this out you can still hang on to the odd pint or three of beer. The key to the whole thing is more activity. It's like you can adjust the thermostat in your house by simply twisting a knob and suddenly your house gets warmer as you use up more heat. You can adjust the thermostat in your body so that you burn up more calories of fat by exercise. But if you try and do it just by dieting, the body will resist it and burn them slower. As for the food cake, it's more about reminding you to include all the things you need than telling you to cut things out. Just use it in whatever way is useful to you.'

'You know, Pete, the thing that gets me is that I'm not much more than a stone and a half heavier than I used to be. But I look at least three and a half stone overweight.'

'It's more a question of overfat than overweight,' I told him. If you're five pounds overweight, you're probably thirteen pounds overfat. People who are just starting to get overweight are already overfat. Fat can be hidden inside the body so that you can be carrying it without seeming overweight at all. You and Ben were once very strong and active, with hard muscles, but since you gave up sport your muscles have simply fattened up. You may be the same weight, but now it's fat and it doesn't look so good.'

He nodded.

'If you were slimmer now,' I asked him, 'would you be feeling differently about food and eating?'

'I'm quite good at picturing how things should be and what I want. I can always picture a car long before I buy it. Those visualisation exercises were quite good for me, but Ben was hopeless. He can't even picture his cat. Some people just can't do that sort of thing you know. That's why I think you might tailor some of those exercises a bit and give us a bit more support during the group.'

'I try to include something for everybody,' I told him, 'but none of it's difficult and all of it needs practice before it gets really useful. Have you lost any weight yet?'

'A couple of pounds. But I look different, I have to admit. You know that 'do nothing while you eat' thing that was driving me crazy?'

'Oh, you mean no pizzas when you're watching football?'

'Yes, that. Well, I've discovered that if you do that, you definitely don't eat as much, do you?'

'That's the idea.'

Do not be too timid and squeamish about your actions. All life is an experience.

Ralph Waldo Emerson

'Well, good on you, Pete. But don't tell anybody I said so. I'll deny it.' He winked and gave me a playful push which knocked me into the pile of chairs.

'Before you go, Lewis, what did you make of that bit when everybody was pretending to be their favourite dessert?'

'You mean what do I think of Lisa's description of Ben?' he said sharply.

Lewis could be surprisingly perceptive.

'Well, I suppose, now you mention it, it was a bit over the top,' I muttered.

'Silly girl, she's wasting her time.' And he was gone.

Chapter 7

Designer Drinking

The days were starting to get longer and riding home along the towpath on the days when I didn't have a late class was a real pleasure. The Tuesday after the evening at the pub, I was almost at the bridge when I overtook another cyclist who was riding a silver mountain bike rather slowly. I called out as I passed, 'Nice bike!'

'Thanks,' came the reply.

I looked over my shoulder to make sure I'd heard what I'd heard. I honestly can't remember what actually happened but the next thing I recall is smelling Chanel No. 5 and realising that I had been right.

When I opened my eyes I appeared to be sitting in the middle of my bike and Lisa had her arm round me. She looked worried but she said, 'You are such a pillock.'

'That's not right, you're meant to ask me if I'm badly hurt. And I'm sure I am.'

'What the hell did you do that for? I only just missed piling into you, and you have no idea how much that bike cost me.'

Typical of Lisa. "Main concern for the fashion accessory," I thought, sadly. 'Actually, I do know how much it cost. I've been wanting one myself. I just can't believe you're riding it.'

'Why shouldn't I? I suppose you think a shopping bike would be more appropriate.'

'Much as I like sitting here in the mud with you, how about helping me out of my bike and we'll have a sensible conversation.'

Lisa stood up and gave me a hand. I was bruised, and the bike wasn't bike shaped anymore. 'You could enter that for the Turner Prize. If you can carry it, why not come back to my place and I'll load it on the roof rack and drive you home. I'll even cook supper for you first.'

That made sense. Lisa and Mo's flat was a lot nearer than mine. 'Thanks Lisa, now tell me when you took up riding a bike?'

'Well, I liked that Sunday afternoon ride and it made me think if I got a proper bike and a helmet that fitted, I might give it a go. And, before you say anything else, let me just say "I told you so".'

The thing always happens that you really believe in, and the belief in a thing makes it happen

Frank Lloyd Wright

'Told me so what?'

'Ages ago, I told you that for all your telling me I've got to stop dieting and start living my life positively, you never believed I could do it. And if you didn't believe I could do it, how was I supposed to believe I could do it?'

'Has it ever occurred to you, Lisa, that once you've convinced yourself you're a failure, you then set about convincing everybody else. And you can be very persuasive. If you really want to change you've got to be prepared to challenge your own beliefs first, and then other people will just follow suit and see you as you see yourself.'

'What?'

'In order to change we have to challenge those beliefs we still live by but which don't work for us any more. Like, in your case, 'I'm overweight,' 'I don't enjoy exercise,' I never stick to an eating plan,' 'I'm never going to be really attractive and successful.' None of those are true, but you've lived by them for as long as I've known you so I suppose you've sold them to me as well as yourself.'

'That statement goes straight in the "Too Difficult" box. We'll talk about it later. I was just making the point that I think you see me as an airhead whose life is out of control.'

'Oh, I never thought you were an airhead. But don't blame me for buying the image you've been selling me for as long as I've known you. You have to convince yourself before you can convince anybody else of anything. Anyway, tell me about the new image, or lifestyle, or whatever it is. How does it feel?'

'It feels funny. Riding to work with a helmet on doesn't exactly fit with my image. My hair's a mess and my mascara runs.'

'So what do you do about that?'

'We've got a company subscription to the Fitness Centre round the corner from my office, so I call in there and do a mini workout and then shower and get ready and walk back to work. In the evening it's OK because I don't have to ride that fast so I don't need to shower all over again.'

'Are you really asking me to have dinner with you when you haven't showered?'

'It's just dinner, Pete.' She looked at me sideways. 'No, actually, I have got an ulterior motive.'

Maybe it wasn't going to be such a bad end to the day after all I thought.

'I want to ask you a favour. Will you run through "Think Before You Eat" with me?' She caught my expression and laughed. 'Honestly, you're as bad as Lewis. Whatever did you think I was going to ask?'

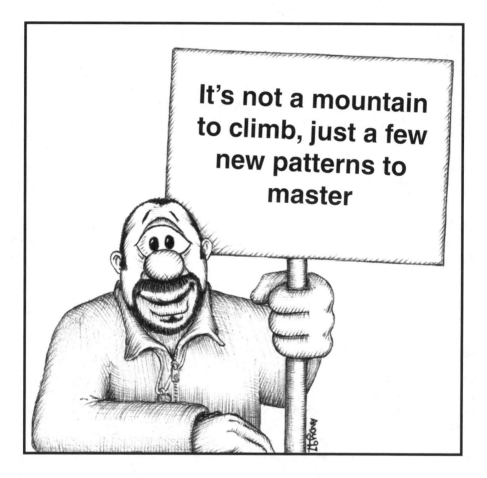

We arrived at the flat and I dumped my bike inside the front gate. 'Not much point in locking it up. Shall I get started in the kitchen while you're putting a mega alarm system on that flashy machine? How much is it insured for?'

She ignored that. 'Just have a look in the fridge and see what there is, I'll be right with you.' It seemed like ages before she reappeared in the kitchen. She looked casually perfect. If I hadn't seen her fifteen minutes earlier looking smudged and dishevelled, I'd never have understood why it took that long to lock up a bike. Still, credit where credit's due, I thought. 'That's a pretty good result for a few minutes effort,' I said. 'but I wouldn't have minded you staying as you were.'

Lisa smiled. 'Thanks, but Ben said he might stop by later.'

'Ben? You're going out with Ben?'

'Don't jump to conclusions. Not yet, we're just thinking about it. He's very attractive.'

'He's as glamorous as that mountain bike.'

'Don't take that analogy any further, please. What shall we eat?'

'Alright Lisa. How hungry are you? What does your stomach feel like?'

'It feels empty, really empty, a bit kind of acid. Usually I have something to nibble while I'm preparing dinner so I don't think about it.'

'So what would feel good inside your stomach at this moment?'

Lisa sat down at the kitchen table and stretched. 'You are so single minded, aren't you? Have we got to do "Think Before You Eat" right now?'

'Well there's not much point in doing it after dinner, is there?'

'I suppose not.'

'Let's get on then. What would feel good inside your stomach?'

She leaned her head back against the wall and looked up at the shelf full of diet books. Suddenly she got up and ran out of the kitchen. 'Oh, no,' I thought, 'not another fifteen minute make-over.' But she was back almost immediately, with an armful of carrier bags.

'I knew the carrier bag collection would come in handy sooner or later,' she said and walked round the table towards me.

'What are you going to do? Haven't I suffered enough already today?' I moved back against the kitchen units. Her expression made me nervous.

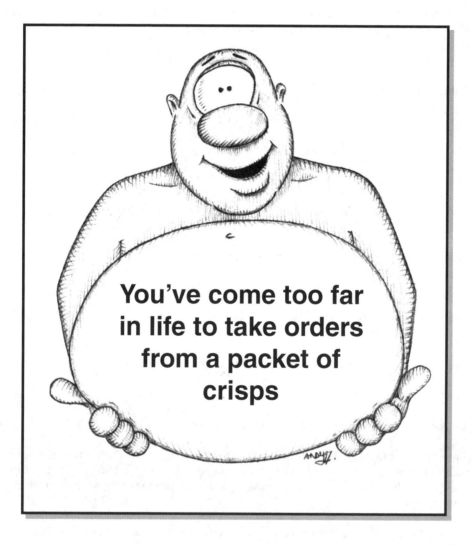

'Just move over, will you.' Lisa pushed past me. If I hadn't stood aside she'd have walked right over me. She started pulling the books off the shelf and dumping them into carrier bags. 'There's a jumble sale at St Mark's on Saturday. These are my contribution to the book stall.'

'What, all of them?'

'All of them. Somebody else can take on my suffering at 10p a go. When I think what I spent on that lot I could weep.'

'I wish I could put all my problems in a carrier bag and give them to a jumble sale.' We both looked round. Ben was standing in the doorway.

'How the hell did you get in?' Lisa asked him.

'The door was open, I called out, but I could hear all this crashing and banging going on in the kitchen so I thought I'd better come down and see if you were all right.'

'Sorry, I probably didn't close the door properly,' I admitted. 'I was feeling pretty shaky, I needed to sit down.' My bid for sympathy didn't even get noticed.

'It's alright,' said Lisa. I could see her looking wildly around the kitchen for a mirror to check her appearance. I've seen that look before.

'You still look great,' I told her. Ben looked at me strangely, then he walked across the room and took the books from Lisa. 'You'll need to double bag these or they'll split,' he told her. 'Where do you want me to put them?'

'By the door. I'll take them round after dinner.'

I suddenly remembered. 'St Mark's won't be open. They're closed for refurbishing till Friday. That's why Miriam set up shop at the Club. I think the jumble sale is their idea of a grand opening ceremony.'

'Oh,' Lisa looked deflated. 'I really wanted to get rid of them right away. It's symbolic.'

'Don't worry,' said Ben, 'let me take them. I've got the car here and I'll just dump them at the school for the Easter Fair. The sixth formers will probably buy them.'

'Poor kids. As if they haven't got enough problems at seventeen.' Lisa commented. 'But, thanks Ben. Why don't you stay to dinner?'

'No dinner till you've finished "Think Before You Eat",' I reminded her. 'And if that fuss over the books was an attempt to distract me, it won't work.'

Ben laughed. 'You should know by now that you can't distract Pete once he's decided to do something. Let's give the man some respect. Hear me now, Lisa, I'll sit right down and do the exercise with you. Go for it, Mr Cohen.'

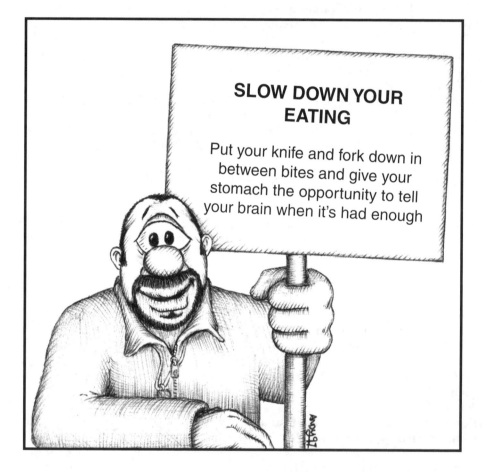

I sat down and faced them both. 'What would feel good in your respective stomachs?'

'Well, I had a very virtuous lunch,' Lisa said. 'Bean salad with tomatoes, onions and some crispbread. I think I fancy some chips and… how about grilled fish? There should be some in the freezer.'

Ben thought for a bit. 'A lamb balti with rice and a couple of cans of Red Stripe to wash it down.'

'Well, apart from the fact that you appear to be incompatible,' I pointed out, 'you now have to think again about those choices and tell me how that food would feel and taste and smell when you're actually eating it. Then, think about afterwards, one hour, maybe two hours later. What's it going to look like in your stomach, what's it going to feel like?'

Lisa put her head in her hands and looked down at the table. 'The chips taste greasy, they feel greasy… I've gone off the idea.'

Ben was frowning. 'I can taste the spices, the sauce, the rice, it still feels good. I admit that it tends to give me heartburn later, but I love it at the time.'

'Try again,' I told them. 'Come up with another choice.'

'Something comforting then,' said Lisa, 'soup, maybe and some really chunky bread.'

'Something hot and spicy, but maybe not quite so fiery, something that would taste good but stay good inside me,' suggested Ben.

'Well, we could go on like this for quite a while,' I said, 'but, for purely selfish reasons, let's compromise. I've had a good look round your fridge, your freezer and all the cupboards, Lisa. All I can find is half a pack of out of date croissants, a lot of un-labelled, unidentified leftovers and some very wrinkly apples. Even the chefs on that TV programme would have trouble making a meal out of it. Here's a suggestion. An Indian takeaway.' I went to stand up but had to sit down again quickly.

Ben said suddenly, 'Are you alright, Pete? You don't look well.'

'I'm shaken and hungry. I fell off my bike. It was Lisa's fault.'

Ben looked confused again. Then he said, 'Let's phone through the order and I'll fetch it. What about some vegetarian stuff? You like that, don't you? Dhal's kind of soupy and comforting. And some rice. How about it?'

The kitchen was quiet while all three of us did a test run on the takeaway. I could see from Lisa's face that she liked it too. And Indian food's my favourite anyway. So it was an easy one.

We had the plates heated and on the table by the time Ben returned. He made sure Lisa and I had taken what we wanted before he filled his own plate.

WATER

Water is an essential part of our bodily needs, second only to oxygen.

Drink 2 – 3 litres of pure water a day.

'You don't have to wait till last,' Lisa said to him. 'Why don't you just dig in?'

Ben looked sheepish. 'I always try and start after everybody else. I eat so fast, I always finish first anyway and then I start picking at what's left on the table. I just can't help it.'

'Have you ever tried to eat more slowly?'

'It's not possible, once I start. My family – we're all that way. If you didn't keep your head down at mealtimes in our house, you missed out. And my auntie, she had a rule about no talking while you're eating.'

'Try putting your knife and fork down between each mouthful,' I suggested.

Ben and Lisa both looked at me as if I was mad.

'Just try it.'

'This is weird,' said Lisa, after a few mouthfuls.

Ben agreed with her. 'I can't go on like this, man, I could die of starvation.'

'Worry about that one if it happens,' I said. 'Just keep doing it. You could try telling a joke between each bite.'

Ben lifted a forkful of rice to his mouth and then put the fork down again, carefully, on the table. 'I don't know that many jokes. Anyway Pete, what does this do for you apart from slowing you down?'

'It makes it easier to taste what you're eating properly and it gives your body time to tell you when you're getting full.'

'What if the food gets cold?' asked Lisa.

'Just take a little at a time and leave the rest on the hot plate.'

Afterwards, I asked them what they thought.

'Actually, after a while, I was doing it automatically and it didn't feel so difficult,' said Ben. 'I could get used to it. And it was good to finish at the same time as you guys instead of sitting watching you for ten minutes.'

'I didn't eat as much as I normally would,' Lisa admitted. 'I definitely knew when I was full. Interesting.'

We sat and chatted for a while until I noticed Ben and Lisa looking at each other. 'Better do the right thing,' I thought. I stood up. This time it felt fine. 'I have to be in early tomorrow, I need to get moving. I can collect my bike tomorrow, Lisa. You don't have to take me back right now.'

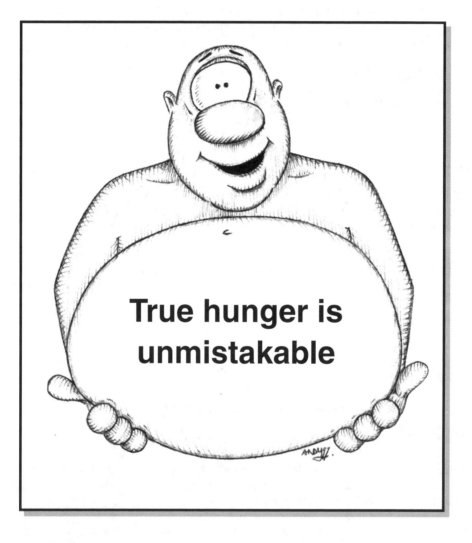

True hunger is unmistakable

'I'll run you home first, and your bike as well,' said Ben. 'You don't look like you should be out walking on the street.' He turned to Lisa who was looking disappointed. 'You come too, and then we can stop for a drink at the wine bar on the way back?'

Just then, Mo arrived. She looked flushed and happy. She gave me a hug and smiled at Ben, then she dived for the fridge door. 'I want something… but what?'

'Well you haven't got much choice apparently,' Ben told her. 'We just had a takeaway.'

'Maybe some fruit.' Mo was still rummaging round the kitchen.

Just then Lisa came back in. 'Hi, Mo. Haven't you had dinner yet? We could have saved you some.'

'Yes, I had dinner already – with Chris before the show.'

'Were you drinking wine? Alcohol dehydrates you. Maybe you're just thirsty,' I suggested.

'I think I'm hungry. How would I know?'

'If you're not sure, there are two ways of finding out. First, have a drink of water and wait a while. Second, run through "Think Before You Eat".'

'We did that before dinner,' Ben told her. 'It was a bit complicated because there were two of us and we thought we wanted different things.' He turned to me, 'Hey, Pete, how did you persuade us we both wanted the same thing which was the same as you wanted? That was either clever or devious.'

I ignored that.

'Well,' said Lisa to Mo, 'if you had dinner a couple of hours ago, you're probably thirsty rather than hungry. It's a good idea to drink a lot of water anyway, I always carry a bottle around with me.'

'Only because it's a fashion accessory right now. You never used to.'

Lisa frowned. 'I'm really fed up with everybody implying that my whole life is some kind of empty fashion statement with no kind of meaning or value whatsoever. Let me tell you all, right now, I sometimes do things because I want to do them. If they happen to be fashionable as well, so what? Anyway, most people don't drink enough water.'

I had to say my bit. 'Lisa's right about that, it's a good idea to drink two or three litres a day. Health and fashion do overlap occasionally.'

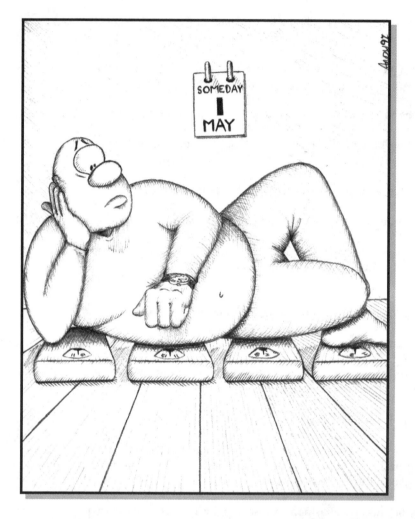

Weight No Longer

'I'd be waterlogged if I drank that much,' Mo protested. 'I haven't got time to spend all day in the loo. Anyway, fashion gets justified by health propaganda too. Thin is meant to be healthy as well as beautiful but you're always going on about how it's not a good idea to be too thin.'

'It depends on how thin and where and what your blueprint is,' I reminded her.

'Remember that conversation we were having,' Mo added, 'about how women always lose weight from their busts first.'

Lisa was relaxing again. She winked at me and said, 'Perhaps I'll just get myself a Wonderbra then, or, better still, go for implants.'

Ben looked alarmed. 'Women were never meant to look like men. I remember my big sister tried to get into my jeans to go to a party. We were the same height when I was fourteen. The waist was too big and the hips were too small and I was so pleased she couldn't wear them because I'd spent all my money on them. I think it was the first pair my auntie didn't buy me. I prefer women to look more natural.'

It was Lisa's turn to be worried. 'That's a really classic male line, I must say. I don't care what most men say, when it comes to the crunch, they go for the Barbie doll every time. Look at the women who get chosen by rich and famous men, I mean men who have a choice. Do they look natural? I don't think so.'

'Actually,' said Mo, 'I didn't have any trouble getting boyfriends before I started losing weight.'

'If that's the case, why are you going to Pete's classes and passing over the creme eggs all of a sudden?' asked Lisa.

'I was actually getting fatter than I was comfortable about. My clothes weren't fitting any more. The trouble is, the more I think about whether I'm overweight, the worse I look and the more anxious I get about it.' She looked across at Ben. 'When you stopped playing rugby, what did you do to keep fit?'

'Nothing, for a while. Every winter, regular as clockwork, I used to start running and dieting six weeks before my two weeks back in St Lucia. By the time I got there, I used to look terrible, feel terrible, and my Mum spent the whole time feeding me up because she was so worried about me. You won't believe this Lisa but I can lose so much weight in six weeks that I look ill.'

'That often happens to people who crash diet,' I said. 'They look gaunt and haggard, right?' He nodded. 'The only criterion for most diets and diet groups is weight loss. Unfortunately, while you're losing fat you may also be losing muscle. The problem isn't loss of fat but loss of muscle. People who get skinny too quickly can still be high in fat.'

'Is that really true?' Lisa asked. 'Maybe that's why I usually feel really under the weather when I've managed to lose a lot in a short time.'

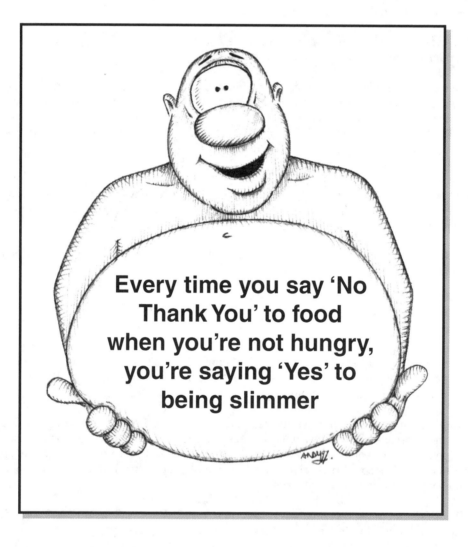

'This all started with me trying to decide whether I'm hungry or thirsty,' Mo reminded us. 'And a lot of help I've had from all of you, Not.'

'Good grief, woman, you're the only person who can decide if you want to eat or drink.'

Mo looked at Ben in surprise. 'That's a funny thing for you to say. And don't call me "woman". Use my name not my category.'

Ben looked thoroughly embarrassed, but he defended himself. 'Well, you were behaving like the kind of silly woman who won't even take responsibility for deciding what she wants or who she is. It's not like you.'

Lisa burst out laughing. 'Actually, it's more like me? Isn't it? No, don't any of you answer that. I'm changing. So, for once, Mo, take some sensible advice from me and drink some water. Ben and I are going out so we'll leave you to it.'

'Well, it's water or nothing if you stay here,' Ben told her. 'You know, Lisa, fashionable or not, I still can't get used to drinking water by itself. It was always tea or orange squash at home and Tizer on holidays. And the drinking fountain in the school playground was enough to put you off completely, unless you wanted a week off sick. Anyway Mo, why don't you come to the wine bar for a late night mineral water with me and Lisa?'

Lisa was looking distinctly put out.

Mo looked at me. 'Are you going too?'

'No, they're dropping me off at home first. I've had a traumatic evening and I need an early night.'

'In that case,' said Mo, 'stay here and keep me company and I'll take you home in half an hour, if you can last that long.'

The relief on Lisa's face was clear. 'Well, if you're both sure, come on Ben, let's go.'

After they'd gone, Mo turned to me and smiled ruefully, 'Aren't we kind, not making gooseberries of ourselves?'

'Do you think that relationship might work?'

'I don't know. I think Ben's a bit too … nice … for Lisa.'

'Hmm. How about you? Where's Chris?'

She looked sad. 'There was a cast party after the performance.'

'Weren't you invited?'

Change your head and the weight loss will follow

'I felt I might be a bit out of place. A lot of the men in that show are slimmer and prettier than me.'

'Oh, I see. Well, have you decided if you're hungry or thirsty?'

'Both. I'm going to have a cup of tea and I've got a secret stash of nuts and raisins. Do you fancy a handful?' She was digging around at the back of the china cupboard.

I started to tell her about what happened on the towpath and she sat down with two mugs of tea and a bowl of dried fruit. A few minutes later she pushed the bowl away and got up. 'I'm not really enjoying them. What do I want?'

'Do you really want anything?'

'Maybe not. You know how it is, you get something to cheer yourself up, you eat it, you don't enjoy it, you feel let down because you didn't get your little shot of pleasure so you look for something else even though by that time you're full up with the stuff you didn't even enjoy.'

'So the snack was just a substitute for Chris, was it?'

'Probably, but actually, just walking through my front door makes me think "food". When I get into the kitchen after a hard day at work, it's just nice to have something to keep you going while you get settled in for the evening, open the post, tidy up a bit, get used to being alone I suppose. I'm used to having people around me at work and our kitchen at home always seemed to be full of people. Having something to eat is almost like having company.'

'Suppose you got into the habit of doing something else instead?'

'Like what?'

'Like maybe lighting some candles, having a bath, doing some stretches and breathing exercises, having a novel on the go and reading a chapter, anything.'

'It sounds much too self indulgent.'

'So what's eating then, if it's not self indulgence?'

'In a way, it's the opposite. You're doing something that tastes good temporarily but even as you taste it you know you're going to feel bad about it and look bad about it later. So it's like Pay As You Earn. Also, you can justify having a biscuit in your hand if somebody turns up unexpectedly but what do I say to my mum if she calls round at 7pm and I'm up to my neck in pink bubbles reading a Mills & Boon?'

'Your mum seemed like a lovely person to me. Wouldn't she understand that?'

'She's a wonderful Jewish mother. She's never done anything in her life that didn't involve looking after other people. Even before she got married she was a nurse. She thinks looking after yourself is immoral. As far as she's concerned at 7pm you should

WALKING YOUR WAY TO SLIMNESS

Anyone can do it

You can do it at your own pace

It's easy

It's enjoyable

It saves bus fares

It burns fat

It will make you fitter

It will get you to where you're going

It's good for the environment

be cooking a proper meal for somebody. She thinks running your own catering business is a poor substitute for having a husband and three lovely children. That's what she had at my age. "Cooking for strangers" she calls my business. Funnily enough, I don't think she would have minded if I'd become a lawyer or a doctor or something. It's just this compromise she can't come to terms with.'

'So you're prepared to live your life according to your mother's belief system?'

'I knew you'd give me a hard time,' said Mo thoughtfully.

'Has she met Chris yet?'

Mo looked alarmed. 'Are you kidding? I don't think she's quite ready for that.'

I thought I'd probably pushed her hard enough. 'Well then, do you want to talk to me about Food Cakes or Pink Elephants, or would you just rather run me and my lump of wreckage home?'

'What a choice. Much as I value your personal attention I think I've had as much insight as I can cope with for one night. Get your bike.'

By Friday the bruising had come out. Most people assumed I'd been in a fight and since that sounded more interesting than falling off your bike I didn't disillusion them. For the first time in ages I was going to hold the group in the River Room, since Miriam had just moved back into St Mark's.

Eve was first to arrive and she immediately spotted the scales and the box of diet milk shakes in the corner. 'I see you've given into tradition at last, Pete. Can I weigh myself first before anybody else gets here?'

'No you bloody well can't. They must be Miriam's, I suppose she forgot them.'

'Alright, alright, calm down Love. What's up with you tonight? Have you had a bad week or something? Oh,' she saw my face as I turned round, 'you have, haven't you. What happened? It wasn't Lewis, was it?'

I felt dreadful for shouting at her. She looked so concerned. 'No, I just fell off my bike, that's all. I'm sorry I snapped at you. But why would you think it was Lewis?'

'I didn't really, it's just that I noticed he keeps challenging you and there's obviously something going on with you and Lewis and Ben and those two girls. You know the short dark one, Mo, she's a funny girl, isn't she?'

'What do you mean, Eve?'

'Well, sometimes, she looks so glamorous, sultry I'd call it, and then another time she'll turn up looking like Waynetta Slob. And what happened to that other woman who used to come with them? She was a strange one as well. Do you know why she dropped out? Not that she really needed to lose weight.'

SETTING YOURSELF UP FOR SUCCESS

How about having outcomes or goals for what you do on a daily or weekly basis?

"I will eat sensibly today"

"I'll eat when I'm hungry"

"I will drink plenty of water"

"I'll exercise today"

Fortunately, before Eve ran out of questions and I had to start trying to come up with answers, Faye turned up. She laid into Eve straight away. 'You didn't call me. You always give me a ring in case I need a lift. Sean couldn't bring me tonight and I've had to walk. I'm all out of breath.'

'I didn't bring the car. I walked too. Don't take on Love. We get brownie points for this.'

'Don't forget to put the pills in the jar,' I said to them. 'It all counts.'

'You know, what?' Faye said. 'It struck me this week, I was thinking about picturing myself slim, not actually doing it you understand, just thinking about it. I was on the bus …'

'You forgot to mention where you were going on the bus, who you sat next to and what you had for breakfast…' Lewis walked past us looking more menacing that usual and sat down.

'Take no notice. One day that young man is going to get his come uppance,' said Eve.

'Don't worry, I think he already has.' Faye was smiling. 'Anyway, what I was going to say was, I couldn't really picture myself slim because I hardly ever have been. I can't really remember what I looked like.'

'Well, when was it, when were you slim?'

'When Sean first started school, I wasn't working then and we didn't have much money, his school was a mile and a half away and it wasn't on the bus route. I just used to walk him there and back. I didn't think about it, there were a lot of other mothers doing the same, and we used to have a chat and a laugh. I must have been walking six miles a day, there and back. I didn't eat any less than I do now, but people used to remark on my figure.'

'They still do,' said Eve.

'Then, when he got old enough to go to school on his own and I started work again, I was going in by train and using the car more at weekends. I don't know, I just went back to being big and buxom. And now, it's really part of my image. I don't know if I can cope with being different.'

I've noticed before that people always tell you important things at impossible times, like when you can't really talk it through with them. I filed it for later. 'Dig out some photos,' I suggested. 'Did you like the way you looked then?'

'I was too busy to think about what I looked like, but I remember feeling a lot better than I've felt before or since. I used to run upstairs, can you believe.'

'Don't despair, Faye. You will run upstairs again. And feel good. Remember the endorphins? Free highs. They're going to start working for you very soon now.'

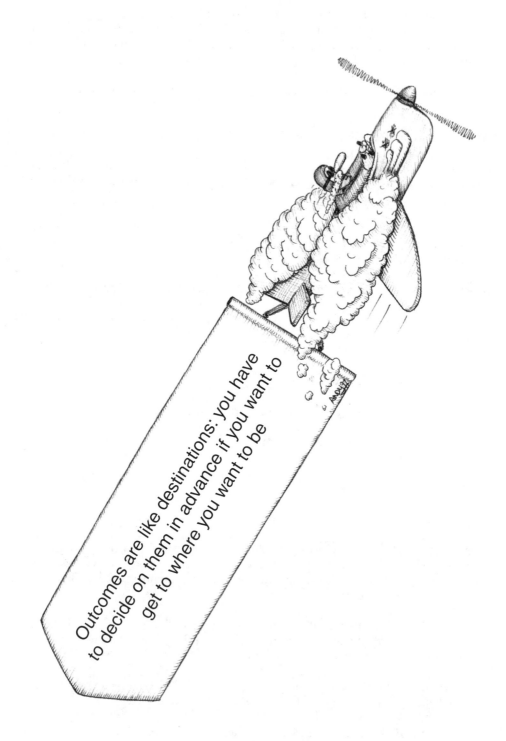

Outcomes are like destinations: you have to decide on them in advance if you want to get to where you want to be

'Oh, yes, they do. I'm a believer. Even now, I'm breathless, but I've got kind of a nice feeling. What I call a bit of a glow. I haven't felt like that since before I got married.'

Eve looked at her sadly. 'I know the feeling. I don't get it very often nowadays. And you know what else, Faye, mind you, Peter's too young to know this ...'

I really hate it when people say that. It's usually something about rationing being good for public health during the war.

Eve continued, 'When you fall in love, you lose your appetite.'

'Better than rationing for losing weight then?' I said, absent mindedly.

'Who said anything about the war?'

'Sorry. Different train of thought. What you're talking about is the endorphin effect again, Eve. Endorphins are natural appetite regulators. And actually, I don't know that falling in love generates them, just like exercise.'

'I know which I'd rather have.' Mo had arrived, out of breath. Lisa was close behind her.

'You can have both,' I suggested. 'Go for it all. Why not.'

By this time, everybody had arrived, so I got them started. 'This evening, we are going to set an outcome for this particular group meeting. At the end of the group we're going to review where we've got to with our outcomes.'

'Sounds like hard work,' objected Eve.

'No, it's not pressure, it's a pull, not a push. Remember the pink elephant. You tend to move towards whatever you visualise. I want you to get into the habit of doing that at the beginning of the day. Set yourself a goal to achieve, doesn't matter how small it is, just a goal you can reach. For example, how about saying to yourself in the morning, "I will be sure to drink at least 8 glasses of water today." Then, when you achieve it, and every day as you achieve more and more of your goals, you must be sure to give yourself credit. Remember the pat on the back?'

'So, we're choosing goals within our reach and setting ourselves up for success?' suggested Mo. 'What about something like, I won't have a Twix at coffee time?'

'No, that's negative. Remember what the brain does with negatives? What happens when you say that to yourself?'

'I fantasise about eating a Twix of course.'

'And is that helpful?'

'No.'

FRUIT AND VEG

Fruit and veggies play an important part in a balanced diet. They are full of vitamins and minerals and they are really good for you.

Consciously make the effort to include more of them in your daily diet.

'Well, don't do it then. Why not go for something positive like: "I'm going to eat when I'm hungry and I'll make sure I have some fruit." Now, how about some ideas from you all for tonight. What do you all want to get out of this evening?'

Lewis stood up and walked to the front, waving some sheets of paper. 'I've got a bone to pick with you about the Food Cake. My objective for this evening is to sort out what I'm meant to be eating. Can I borrow the flip chart?'

'Be my guest.' I was really quite nervous. I had the session pretty carefully planned and I hadn't included a guest speaker. As if I hadn't had enough the door then opened again and in came Chris, dressed to kill. Personally, I've never understood how women can walk in high heels, never mind men. He swayed into the nearest empty seat which was next to Ben. I saw Ben look at him curiously and then turn back to watch what Lewis was doing.

Lewis drew a circle and filled in the sections very quickly and accurately.

'That's clever,' commented Lisa. 'I thought you were a programmer, not an artist.'

He smiled at her and there was one of those four-second blips in the room that feels like forever.

'What's the point you're making, Lewis?' I asked him.

'Well, look at it, will you, that's a typical day for me. That's how I eat. That's what I like eating.'

We all focused our attention on the chart.

The fruit and vegetable side was rather blank. One piece of fruit was filled in and two vegetables, but the other side was a different story. He'd added three or four extra slices of bread, doubled the fat, trebled the fish/meat section and increased the sugar.

'Well, that explains it,' said Faye.

'Explains what?'

'Why you can't lose weight. I'm surprised you aren't two stone heavier.'

'Did you ever think about what you ate before, Lewis?'

'Not really. I always thought I had a pretty good diet, I don't eat sweets or cakes or anything like that.'

'So where did all the fat and sugar come from?'

I think,
therefore I am

René Descartes

'I got into high energy drinks when I was training and I usually have a can of coke on the go while I'm working. And on my way into work in the morning I pick up a bacon and egg sandwich. I like chips. I like sugar in my tea, butter on my bread … and I've never liked green vegetables. I'll eat vegetable soup or a stew or something but Brussels sprouts make me feel ill just to think about.'

'The Food Cake is a continuation of the Food Diary. The idea is to make you more aware of what you're actually eating and how that measures up to what you really need.'

'I don't see the point of knowing how much crappy food I eat if I can't do anything about it.' He turned to go back to his seat, noticed Chris had taken it and, suddenly, Lisa smiled at him again. Twice in one evening, I thought. He headed for the seat next to her, knocking down a chair and stepping on Eve's toes to get there.

I relaxed. 'Knowing what you're eating is just the first step to making changes. You can't change something you don't know about. What I suggest you do is add an extra serving of some kind of vegetable every week. Do you like carrots?' Lewis nodded. What about salad?' He nodded again. 'There you are then, you can all make small changes, a few at a time. Some of you will change faster than others but you will all be surprised at just how easily and naturally the right foods will start creeping into your diet and on to your plate if you just let them.'

Faye put her hand up. 'I've started doing that. I can't stand cabbage, but I'm eating more peas and salads. There's always something you can do. I don't think the Food Cake means that everybody has to eat exactly the same.'

'Well,' said Lisa, 'I felt a bit silly colouring in the Food Cake, but it's a really graphic way to see where you need to adjust what you're eating. At a glance in fact, there it is. Whether you like it or not. And I didn't at first.' She turned to Lewis. 'One item at a time, over the weeks, you can make little adjustments.'

Lewis was completely mesmerised.

At the end of the group, I gave them a final exercise to take away. 'Here's another thing I want you to do. Affirmations. Every morning, as well as stating your outcomes for the day, I want you to make an affirmation for yourself. 'I am …' and, throughout the day, get used to repeating it to yourself, over and over.

'How about 'Eagles, Eagles, Eagles,' suggested Ben.

The group turned to him, blankly.

'It's the Crystal Palace chant. If you all did it a hundred times a day, like I do, we might win next Saturday.'

Eve stood on her chair. Come on everybody. 'Eagles, Eagles, Eagles.'

Many diets tell you not to eat certain foods.

You can.

If you're telling yourself what you shouldn't eat, you're actually focusing your mind on it:

I mustn't **EAT CHOCOLATE**

Instead, remind yourself, you have a choice. You can eat what you want. The question is

Do you really want it?

What will it do for you if you eat it?

Are you really hungry?

Is there a more delicious and healthy alternative?

It was quite hypnotic. Everybody who wasn't laughing too much joined in. It was then that Miriam came through the door and stopped on the threshold. I would say she was open mouthed, but Miriam was too much in control of her features to do anything so inelegant.

'Well,' she said, eventually, 'this is some new technique I haven't heard about, obviously. Does chanting burn calories as well as calming the mind? Or have I wandered into the yoga class by mistake?'

'Hello Miriam. Just in time for the pub as usual.'

She smiled, in spite of herself. 'I only came to get the scales and diet drinks.'

'How did your group go without the weigh-in?' I asked her.

'Your sarcasm is wasted on me, Peter. We managed perfectly well. I thought to myself, "If Mr Cohen can do it without scales, so can I."'

'It sounds to me like one of those car stickers,' suggested Chris. 'Dieters Do It Without Weighing The Consequences.'

Chapter 8

When The Going Gets Tough

I decided it was time to have a party to celebrate my new kitchen which was going to be ready the week before Easter. My flat wasn't that big, but, in the end, I invited everybody. Including the current Lighten Up group. Lisa and Mo were friends anyway, but I always feel as though I'm sharing a crucial part of people's lives while a group's actually running. Losing weight, or changing shape, successfully, is a serious life change and rites of passage are required.

It wasn't till Wednesday lunchtime that I settled down during my break to draft the invitations. I wanted to get them copied on the way home.

'What are you doing?' Jane looked over my shoulder.

'It's the grand opening of my refurbished kitchen. Not enough room to swing a cat, but it's being repainted and I'm having a new cooker.'

'Great. Can I come?'

I looked up at her. She didn't look well. In fact, she seemed to have been taking days off here and there for several weeks. Seeing the dentist, food poisoning, 'flu, one thing after another. She used to be one of the most reliable people I'd ever worked with but just lately I'd been covering a lot of her classes for her. 'If you're well enough. Should you be in today?'

'Yes, I'm fine. I'm just going out for a sandwich. Do you want anything?'

'Mmm, I'm definitely hungry, hang on a second…'

Then she snapped. 'Here we go, "What do I want? What do I feel like?" Can't you ever just do something simple like choosing lunch without going through this diet class carry-on? How long is this going to take? – I'm in a hurry.'

I was surprised. She used to be pretty laid back but just lately she seemed to be stressed out about everything. 'It just takes me a second or two, that's all. You might not be off sick quite so often if you paid more heed to your body instead of shoving the first thing down your throat that came to hand. You don't think about what you eat either before you eat it or while you eat it. You should try it my way sometime. You might enjoy it.'

'Don't be so bloody self righteous. I didn't mean to snap at you.'

'OK, no problem. If you're going down to the café, just get me the soup and one of those sunflower rolls with some tomato salad.'

"Have some soup," Lizzie said. "Soup is good for stress."

Marsha Norman

– The Fortune Teller

When she came back I hit 'Save' and swung round in my chair. 'Come and talk to me while we have lunch. You can take ten minutes off to do that.'

She didn't argue and we both went over to the window overlooking the river to eat. I noticed she had bought herself exactly the same as me. 'I may be self-righteous, but I don't expect everybody to eat what I eat. I just noticed they had carrot and orange soup on the board today and that's what I fancied.'

Jane shook her head. 'I just couldn't be bothered to make a decision. Actually, this is nice. How long have they been doing this bread? I usually have the Chef's Special on a baguette but he's been overdoing the garlic lately.'

I remembered Lewis's comment, but I didn't say anything. She was eating like a steam train as usual. 'Slow down, enjoy it. You've got time. Taste it.'

'I've got so much to catch up on. I feel guilty about landing you with so many of my classes. Hang on a minute.' She got up and walked over to her desk, pulled a box of doughnuts out of the top drawer and came back. 'I didn't even think I'd have time for lunch today, so I bought these on the way in. We can have them for pudding. I'll make some coffee.'

'Wait five minutes and see if you still want one. I'll make the coffee. You, sit right there.'

'Why five minutes?'

'Because then you'll know if you're still hungry. If you just carry on eating, you'll miss the point when you're satisfied.'

She raised her eyebrows but didn't argue. When I came back with the coffee she was sitting on the floor, back against the wall, with her eyes closed.

'Here you are. Now, how about a doughnut?'

'Thanks, Pete. No, I don't want one any more. Now, see what you did?'

'What did I do?'

'You stopped me having a treat. And I was looking forward to it. Let me tell you, there are positive aspects to not being as disciplined over food as you are. If I hadn't waited five minutes, I wouldn't have known I wasn't hungry and I would have really enjoyed that one with the chocolate icing.'

'But how would you have felt afterwards?'

'That's not the point. You denied me a little bit of pleasure!'

'I see. Life's so bad at the moment that a doughnut makes all the difference, is it?'

Repetition is the mother of all skill

'Every little escape is worth having. My first exam's this weekend and I just know I'm not going to get the marks I need.'

'Oh, your OU degree? You don't talk about it, so I forget you're doing it. I don't know how you manage to work and study at the same time. Why didn't you ask for study leave?'

Jane twisted her long black ponytail round her fingers. 'I'm sorry, I just couldn't afford it so I took sick leave instead. I couldn't very well tell you because then you'd have been involved, wouldn't you? Anyway, I've been eating so much and not doing so much exercise that now I'm feeling bad about that, as well as everything else. Just look at me. I felt totally embarrassed in the aerobics class this morning.'

She used to look like a gladiator, but I had noticed lately a tendency to wear baggy T shirts a lot. In fact, it was hard to tell what shape she was. 'Why not tackle one thing at a time. You've got to eat. You've got to study. Just tell yourself that the two things are mutually exclusive. When you feel the need to nibble, do something else instead. Get right up, out of your chair and do yourself a little mini exercise routine. That's easy for you.'

'I don't know if I can study without eating. Books and biscuits go together. I've never been good with exams. As soon as I sit down to study I just eat and worry instead. That's why I'm still trying when everybody else has got their qualifications.'

'So books and biscuits are a hard-wired connection. Suppose you break it and make another one instead?'

'What, another connection with biscuits or another connection with books?'

'Forget the biscuits for now. Let's think about the books. What about, when you sit down with your books, always putting on a tape of something you like, preferably without words of course. Just keep a stack of really lively music by you when you're studying and when you want to reach out for a biscuit, reach out for a tape instead. But I'll tell you a secret. There's only one way this strategy will work.'

'How?'

'You have to do it over and over and over and over again. Repetition is the mother of all skill.'

'It's more likely to be the mother of all battles – with myself! I'll give it a go, but the only thing I'll promise is that I won't take any more time off. Now I come to think of it, you're looking a bit tired too.'

Having overrun my lunch break, I needed to catch up. The rest of the day didn't get any better. One of the machines broke down and when I checked through the in-trays there seemed to be endless urgent paperwork. I guessed Jane had been letting it pile up.

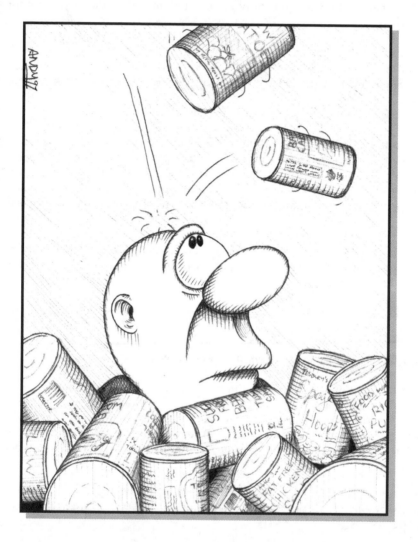

Think Before You Shop

By the time I left, I remembered I had nothing for breakfast and not much of anything else back at the flat. While the kitchen was being fixed I'd been eating out a lot and buying takeaways. Now there was no excuse. So there I was, at ten o' clock on a Wednesday night, pushing my trolley round the supermarket with my list in my hand. I knew exactly what I needed so I was pretty focused. Normally, I just drift around and pick up whatever comes to mind but I was making an effort to live by my own rules so I made sure I only bought what I'd planned to buy in advance. I was concentrating so hard that I didn't even see Ben until we ended up in a Sicilian lock with an enormous woman in camouflage and army boots. His trolley was full of salad and Vimto.

'What are you doing here?' we both asked, as if there was anything else we could be doing. Ben looked even more fed up than me. I looked at the random assortment of people around us. 'Have you noticed how many weirdos you get shopping at this time of night?'

'I think these late night supermarkets were invented to give lost souls a place to go when the sun goes down. And have you noticed what they're buying?' He glanced over his shoulder, 'There is a man over there with a trolley full of Jaffa Cakes. I was talking to somebody the other night who said she often goes late on a Saturday night and it's fruit cake city then.'

'I'm not surprised,' I said. 'It's probably better than sleeping pills. Have you ever noticed how tired you feel when you get home with a pile of groceries? Shopping before bedtime must be a great way of making sure you go to bed tired. And who's "she," by the way?'

Ben looked sheepish. 'Lisa. It was Lisa. We met again last night for a drink after work and I've asked her out for dinner tomorrow. Don't say anything. I don't know if it's a good idea. We're kind of different.'

'I suppose both of you being into weight control is some kind of basis for a relationship,' I said. 'But if you plan to go out for dinner you'd better synchronise your diets first. Better still, why not get the dieting sorted and then you might find some more interesting things to talk about.'

I was a bit nervous about Ben and Lisa getting together. Funnily enough, it wasn't so much Lisa I was concerned about as Ben. Apart from his brief flirtation with dodgy diets, he'd always struck me as rather down-to-earth and sweet-natured, and quite shy. Lisa seemed to have a way of infecting perfectly sensible people with a touch of her own obsessions.

'I don't know where to take her. She can be very picky. Do you have any ideas for me?'

'Take her somewhere expensive where they serve very small, highly decorated portions.'

He nodded. 'That's a good idea. I sometimes think she's afraid of food.'

THINK BEFORE
YOU SHOP

When you go shopping:

Ask yourself what food you need to have in store and what meals you want to eat

Read the labels and choose foods that have a high nutritional value

Shop more often and buy fresh foods, particularly fruit and vegetables

Watch out for hidden fat and sugar

Look to cut down on E numbers

Buy a good balance and variety of foods

'I'm not surprised. Most dieters are one bite from failure and she's a professional dieter.'

Ben shrugged. 'I wouldn't have understood that five years ago, but you know what? Towards the end of my food combining period I was starting to get stressed out unless I could eat the right stuff at exactly the right time. That kind of thing can take over your life.'

I decided to change the subject. 'Did everybody come round for the football tonight?'

'Oh yes, man, they certainly did. And where were you?'

'Running Jane's evening sessions. She's been having a lot of 'flu lately.'

'I remember her. So garlic doesn't work.'

I looked at him carefully. He was quite straightfaced. In fact he looked as if his mind was somewhere else.

'I tell you something though,' he said suddenly, 'We did not order pizzas this time. Or last week.'

'I know. Lewis was making a big fuss about it in the group, remember?'

Ben continued. 'I thought you were right about not just sitting there in front of the box eating stuff we weren't even tasting. Plus, I've been filling in the Food Cake which focuses my mind quite a lot. It's just so graphic, you can't help seeing what you're missing out on. But, see, I have this problem.' He leaned towards me, and put his hand on my shoulder. I tensed, I don't know why. But I needn't have worried.

'Since I gave up my food combining,' Ben whispered, 'I sometimes find myself in the fried chicken shop on the way home from work. I don't mean to do it, but fast food just happens to me sometimes when I'm tired and my resistance is low.'

I laughed. Ben was indignant. 'What's funny about it?'

'With that build up I thought it was going to be drugs or sex. At least. And don't worry about the fried chicken, it's the smell. It goes straight to your hypothalamus.'

'What?'

'Never mind. What did you and the lads do while you were watching the game then?'

'We met straight after work and went out for a curry early on. Remember that night I called round at Lisa's flat and we had a curry? Well, we went to the same place and ate in. I had a tandoori which is not bad when I usually have a korma, you know, all the cream and so on. I was proud of myself. After that we walked back to my place, and that's not all. We walked down to the pub and back afterwards. In fact, that's where I've just come from. They're all still there.'

CLUES FOR READING LABELS

If it has a scientific name, it's usually man-made and is an E number.

Nutritional value is measured in:

> Protein
> Fat
> Carbohydrates (simple and complex)
> Minerals and vitamins.

If a label doesn't have calorific values on it, remember that any fat has 9 calories per gram but protein and carbohydrate only have 4 calories per gram.

Really cheap items are usually composed largely of chemicals and the name of the product (pizza, bread...) may be the only thing you recognise on the label.

Don't look for perfection, go for balance and variety from different food groups.

It's one step at a time, I thought. Walking to the pub is better than sitting drinking beer at home. At least he's thinking about it. I couldn't resist commenting on his trolley. 'Is this the latest eating plan?'

He laughed. 'You can't complain about the salad. And I still prefer Vimto to all this designer water.'

We were passing the tinned food now and he automatically reached out for a steak and kidney pudding. 'Do you ever read labels?' I asked him.

'Of course I read labels. That's how I know it's mince. And I always buy the big name brands because my auntie used to tell me the stores Own Brands use inferior ingredients. They're like cheap imitations of the real thing. I don't mind paying a few extra pence if I know I'm buying a reputable brand.'

'I mean the small print. Do you actually check what's in those cans?'

'Mince of course.'

'Why not read it and see.' I grabbed a can from him. 'I heard recently that a tin of this stuff had less than half beef in it. The rest was cereal and mechanically recovered chicken.'

Ben looked appalled. He snatched the can back and read out the ingredients. '"Water, wheatflour, beef, pork, kidney, beef fat, rusk, salt, raising agents, malic acid, sodium bicarbonate, yeast extract, colours, caramel, pepper, onion extract, E202 ..." Hey, what is all this stuff?'

'Well you've got a few chemicals in there. And, before you ask, there isn't a section for them on the Food Cake. In my opinion you don't need them. Why don't you just buy fresh food?'

'It means I have to shop more often, and it takes longer to cook.' He started laughing. 'Get out of here, you interfering bastard. You just ruined my evening. I'm not going to get back before closing time if I have to read all the labels.' He abandoned the tinned food and headed for the bakery section. I left him debating about wholemeal versus granary: 'Wholemeal tastes like sawdust but the granary gets in your teeth.'

Friday night I was getting ready for the group when Faye turned up, early. She looked terrible. I felt I knew her well enough by now, so I put my arm round her. 'How are your outcomes, Faye?'

She burst into tears. She hadn't done that since that telephone conversation after the first class. 'You know I try to be a positive sort of person, Pete, but I feel so bad.'

'Why?'

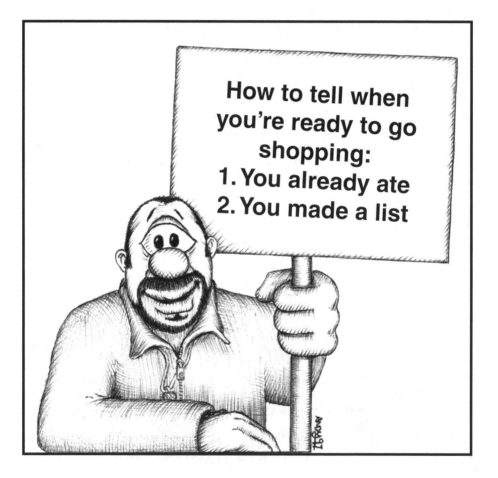

'I'd been having a really good week. I'd been setting myself goals every day. I'd been deciding at the beginning of each day what were the outcomes I wanted, all lovely positive ones. Then, I set myself this outcome yesterday, I was going to take two Fat Burning Pills, ride my bike to work and do the last day of the Food Cake. I always think my outcomes through while I'm getting my face on in the morning. Well, I went downstairs, feeling pretty positive, picked up the post and made a cup of tea. The first thing I open is this letter from the bank manager. He's telling me I'm overdrawn and at first I can't think why and then I remember. I know I asked Sean to get some money out on my cash card for me Monday night and he must have met his father. They took out the maximum amount, all in one go. He just gave me the twenty I'd asked for and I never thought any more about it. I get this funny feeling in my chest sometimes and I could feel it then so I opened the freezer and heated up a whole pack of croissants. I ate the whole lot and I was late for work as well. I felt terrible for the rest of the day.'

'Listen, Faye, we can sort this out. Come for a drink with me after the class, just the two of us. Jane's doing the aerobics for me this week and I've got some ideas you can use in this sort of situation.'

She'd recovered a bit by the time everybody else arrived. 'Did the Palace win last Saturday?' she asked Ben, as he sat down next to her.

'If you ask me, everybody had their mind on chanting for their own selfish purposes,' he told her. 'If you had all done as I suggested we would not have been humiliated again.'

Lisa came in then and sat next to Ben on the other side. 'What were you saying to the mirror every morning? Don't tell me you were really going 'up the birds' or whatever. I bet you were going 'I am slim and fit,' just like the rest of us.'

He smiled. But I couldn't see any sign of rapport between them. I wondered how the dinner date had been.

After the class, I went over to Faye and told her to meet me at the Café Rouge. 'Better avoid the Duke's Head, everybody else will be there.'

'I'll get you a drink,' she said and slipped out while the others were still talking.

Lisa walked over. 'Thanks for the party invitation, Pete. I'd love to come. Do you want some help with the food? Mo and I could come over for the afternoon and give you a hand.'

'If you could help me with the shopping that would be even better. No sooner do I get the kitchen fixed up than the car breaks down. Just as long as you don't want to do it last thing at night or something.'

'Oh, Ben told you about that, did he?'

'What were you doing at the supermarket on a Saturday night?'

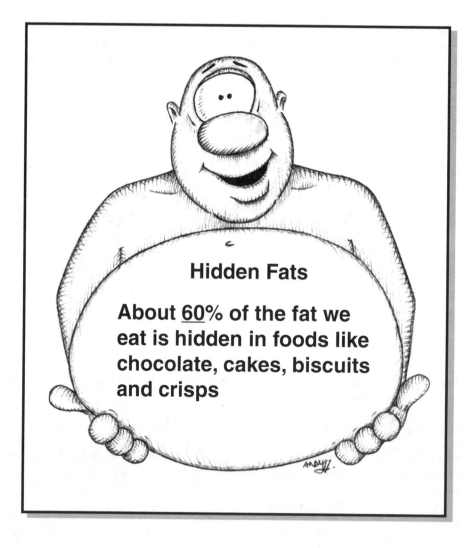

Hidden Fats

About <u>60</u>% of the fat we eat is hidden in foods like chocolate, cakes, biscuits and crisps

'I just knew I wouldn't be able to sleep and I'd had enough exercise even for me that day. And we needed some basics. It was a disaster though. The shop wasn't very busy and as I didn't have anything else to do except go home to sleep, which I couldn't, I just drifted around loading junk into the trolley.'

'No list?'

'No list. Usually I go with Mo and she's really organised. Because she has to be for her business I suppose. She knows what she wants and how much. And we always make sure we've had dinner before we go. You know the old saying, "don't go shopping when you're hungry," well, it makes sense. But that night, I blew all the rules. Mind you, I did sleep well afterwards, but I had to invite a few people round for drinks the next day to take care of all the popcorn and peanuts. I didn't dare leave them lying about at home.'

'Where is Mo, by the way?' I was looking over her shoulder. This group was certainly bonding. They were in a huddle, obviously planning the rest of the evening.

'She's in the middle of that lot, with Chris probably. Did you notice, he's done it again?'

'What, come as the wrong gender?'

'Yes. And I bet he's going to come to the pub like it as well.'

'Be reasonable, Lisa. He can hardly change mid-evening, can he? Where would he do it, the Gents or the Ladies? Anyway, he usually goes back to work after the class, doesn't he?'

'The show's finished its run so he's at a loose end until next week. Then he's got another booking that takes him through Easter. I'll say this for him, he doesn't spend much time resting. Anyway, I must go. Are you coming to the Duke's Head or are you sneaking off with Faye?'

'I promised I'd run through something with her, but we'll join you all later.'

When I got to Café Rouge, Faye was sitting in a corner with a cappuccino in front of her. She pushed my mineral water towards me as I sat down. I noticed that when she was unhappy she looked much older. Normally she was one of those people who seemed pretty much ageless.

'I'm sorry,' was the first thing she said. 'The last thing you want is to spend your Friday evening talking to me. You should be over at the Duke's Head with the other young people.'

'Stop apologising. It doesn't suit you. I'm experimenting on you anyway so it works both ways.'

'Experimenting. I like the sound of that. If the experiment works will I be rich, thin and happy for the rest of my life?'

HOW TO REDUCE THE FAT YOU EAT

Use skimmed or low fat milk, non-fat or low fat yoghurt

- Eat less meat, eat leaner meat, remove fat and skin and limit processed meat

- Eat plenty of fruits and vegetables

- Eat whole grain bread

- Use non-stick pans and sprays for cooking

- Substitute low fat or non fat plain yogurt for sour cream or mayonnaise

- Grill or bake meat instead of frying

- Eat more fish – it's low in saturated fat, cholesterol and calories and it's a good source of protein, B vitamins and zinc

'If I could figure out a way of doing that for people in half an hour I could get my car fixed and retire to Grand Cayman. Now, that rough patch you went through yesterday. Let's run through it again.'

'I don't want to. It was bad enough the first time.'

'This is a trial run for the next disaster that might sneak up on you before breakfast and sabotage your outcomes. Now, what were those outcomes you'd decided on?'

'Take two Fat Burning Pills, ride my bike to work and fill in my Food Cake down to the last greasy crumb.'

I looked at her sternly.

'Alright, down to the last slice of apple.'

'That's better. Now, you've got your face on, you've got your outcomes, you've made it down the stairs. You pick up the letter and head for the kitchen, open the letter and you're straight into the danger zone. The lure of the croissants is almost overwhelming, you want to blot out the letter, right? You need a fast hit of something wicked enough to take the pain away?'

'Yes, I'm on the brink of disaster. My resistance is low.'

'Right, this is where I intervene. You open the freezer door. You take out the croissants. They're in the oven. You're starting to smell them. What are you doing while you're waiting?'

'Getting the jam and butter out.'

'And are you feeling good?'

'No, I'm feeling wretched. But I know I'll feel better when I'm actually eating them.'

'While you're waiting for those croissants, try this. Try feeling really bad and see what happens.'

Faye stared at me. 'You are mad. You're absolutely barking. I'm only eating the croissants because I'm trying to make myself feel better.'

'Exactly. And does it work? For how long? Minutes? Seconds? Or are you feeling bad about eating them while you're actually eating them? You're going to feel bad anyway, so why the hell don't you get it over with by feeling bad about the original problem? You should have felt bad. What happened was upsetting to say the least. But what did you do? Instead of taking the hit and getting angry with Sean and his father, you ate some croissants and ruined your whole day. Your whole day. What had you done wrong? Nothing. You didn't deserve that.'

Tears were rolling silently down Faye's cheeks. 'I can't bear it.' Was all she could say.

If you are distressed by anything external, the pain is not due to the thing itself, but to your estimate of it; and this you have the power to revoke at any moment.

Marcus Aurelius

'Yes you can. You're, what, fifty quid down? A hundred? I don't want to know. But it won't happen again because this time, you've faced it. Now, let's start yesterday again. This time, you can eat the croissants. On the condition that you've allowed yourself to feel the pain and anger first.'

'Wait a minute, I thought we were going to do it without me eating the croissants.'

'You can't put the clock back. Eat them. Enjoy them. Or not, as the case may be. Maybe you won't want to eat them all this time. But it doesn't matter. When you've finished eating, leave the plates right where they are and go back upstairs to fix your face again.'

'Oh, but I didn't need to… yes… I do need to… My God, Pete, what day is it?' She shot off to the Ladies and I settled down to my pint and the Standard crossword. I didn't look up when she slipped back into the seat beside me. 'Feel free to get angry with me, if you like,' I said. I was afraid to look up.

'Angry about what?' said Mo.

I looked up. Mo was sitting where Faye had been. 'I thought you were Faye. She's just gone to the loo.'

'Is she having problems?'

'She certainly is. But nothing that can't be solved.'

'And you're giving her a bit of free counselling?'

'Nope. I'm not qualified to do that. I was just telling Faye that if you apply the wrong remedy to a problem, you can make the situation worse. Food, for example, doesn't cure emotional pain. It just gives you something else to worry about. In my opinion it's better to try and solve the real cause of the unhappiness than to add more weight to the problem.'

Mo nodded. 'Trying to fill an emotional hole with food. It doesn't work, does it?'

Before I could reply, Faye re-appeared. She'd done a pretty good job with her face. Mo stood up and said, 'I'll go, I just came to see if you two were going to join the rest of us.'

Faye grabbed her arm. 'No, stay for a minute. I don't mind telling you what happened and then we can all walk over together, but I've got to finish what we started. Just to fill you in, Mo, I got upset about something, had a blast of comfort-eating and blew all my outcomes for the day completely out of the water.'

'That is one of my all-time favourite behaviour patterns,' said Mo. 'Been there, done that. How about sharing the solution with me?'

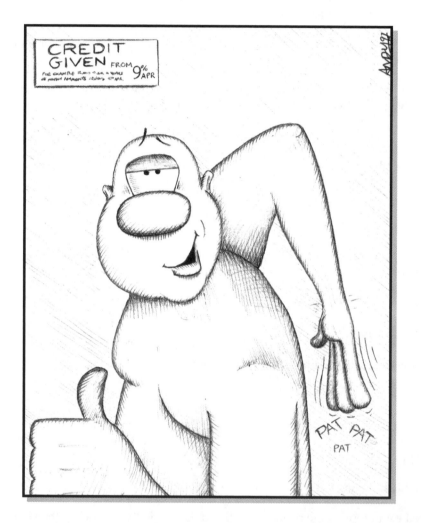

When you're triggered to eat for any reason apart from hunger, and you do something else instead, give yourself some credit

'Alright,' Faye continued, 'that's what Pete's helping me with. Let's get back into yesterday morning. What do I do when I've eaten all the croissants and repaired my make-up?'

'You get on your bike and go to work,' I said. 'And, at lunchtime, you take your first Fat Burning Pill. And, if you're hungry, you get something sensible to eat.'

'What, eat at lunchtime when you've pigged out at breakfast? No way!' Mo and Faye were both outraged.

'What happened at breakfast is over and done with. Just get right back on track with your day and then at least you've still completed the outcomes you set yourself. Just because one thing's gone wrong for you doesn't mean you have to ruin everything else by eating so much that you feel even worse than you did when you started.'

'So I have to fill all the croissants in on the Food Cake? That's adding insult to injury. And what happens next time? Because there's always a next time, isn't there? What then?' asked Faye.

'Next time unhappiness drives you to the biscuit tin, stop and ask yourself what the pain's all about. Let yourself feel the pain for a minute. Honour your feelings for goodness sake. If something awful happens at least respect yourself enough to let yourself feel the pain. Then, when you've come to terms with it and survived it, ask yourself, "Did eating cure this pain last time?" and, if the answer is "no, it made me feel worse" then do something different.'

'I'm not with you,' said Faye. 'Do what different?'

'Well, when you feel bad, instead of eating, do something else. Getting out of the house is often a good idea - move away from the surroundings that trigger the eating. Have a good cry if you have time. Light a candle and meditate for five minutes. Run up and down stairs. Give the cat a cuddle. Phone somebody up. Just try something different.'

'Don't forget your affirmations,' Mo said quietly. 'Several times, in dire circumstances, I've found myself walking round the block going "I'm slim, getting slimmer, I'm fit, getting fitter". The neighbours think you've finally flipped because you're talking to yourself. Which is true of course. But it's amazing what you can convince yourself of if you say it often enough.'

There was silence for a minute. Then Faye stood up. 'Why don't we go and join the others. Do I look alright?'

'You look terrific.'

When we got to the Duke's Head it was packed but I soon spotted the Lighten Up barflies. I could hear them as well. Or Chris at least. He was doing a reasonable imitation of Lisa Stansfield on the Karaoke. Mo's face was a tragedy but Faye grasped the situation immediately and whisked us both out of the door again.

The easiest way to change your body is to eat the highest quality, lowest fat, highest volume food.

Wherever possible go for unprocessed, whole grain products.

Long Grain Brown Rice
Brown Pasta
Potatoes
Wholemeal Bread
Cous Cous
Millet
Buckwheat
Keniou

Faye covered her ears. 'I can't stand Karaoke. My husband used to make me watch his Elvis impressions every Thursday until I dug my heels in and refused. I think that was the beginning of the end of my marriage. Let's go somewhere else.'

'Good idea,' Mo said, bravely. 'How about a pizza?'

Faye hesitated for a moment. 'Did you eat before the class, Mo? And what about you, Pete?'

'Yes, but it was just a bowl of muesli. I didn't have time for anything else. I wouldn't mind something light, and a drink. I've had three glasses of wine already tonight and I'm dehydrated.'

I hadn't eaten since about four o' clock and I knew I'd be walking home as usual. With no car and the insurance company being slow about the bike I was totally without transport. 'I'm up for it, what about you, Faye?'

'My eating's been all over the place since yesterday. I haven't had anything since breakfast.'

'Still punishing yourself?' asked Mo. 'I'm coming to the conclusion that there's no point in giving yourself a hard time when somebody else will usually do it for you free of charge.'

A few minutes later we were in Angelo's. It was easy to get a table because we'd beaten the after-the-pub rush. 'I'm having the salad, and some of that ciabatta with a glass of wine,' Faye announced as she passed the menu on to Mo.

Mo closed the menu and put it on the table in front of her. 'I'll have a pizza but I'm going to impress you both by drinking water with it. I remember you telling us, Pete, that if we feel thirsty the dehydration process is already setting in. I've thought about it and I'm definitely thirsty.'

The meal went better than I'd expected although Mo was a bit hyper, I thought. Faye seemed comfortable with herself and what she was eating. 'How did that feel?' I asked her afterwards.

'Much better. It's nice to take time over a meal, isn't it? Sometimes really simple food just tastes good, especially when you know you aren't going to suffer from an attack of guilt afterwards. Since Thursday morning I've either been eating because I was unhappy or not eating because I was unhappy. My meals haven't had anything to do with being hungry. And, of course, that made me feel worse because I'd pretty much got the hunger scale sorted before that, so I'd been feeling quite pleased with myself.'

'You know, Faye, you've got to start measuring your successes instead of just clocking your failures. Are you giving yourself credit when you do something right? It's not so much your behaviour that's important as your response to it.'

AFFIRMATIONS

Many famous people owe their success to messages they constantly repeated to themselves over and over again. "I am famous, I am rich…"

Make up an affirmation, something that reminds you of what you're doing and makes you feel positive and in control.

I'm becoming strong and slender and nothing stops me.

I'm slim and getting slimmer.

I'm fit and getting fitter.

'What, you mean the patting yourself on the back routine? Sean caught me doing that Tuesday night and I had to tell him I'd swallowed something the wrong way.'

'So do you think you can get back to eating and drinking when your body asks for it again?'

'Yes, I think so. It's just a question of getting things in perspective, isn't it? After all, I've got plenty of evidence that eating and drinking when you're not hungry doesn't make you feel good. So why do I keep doing it?'

'I suppose,' said Mo, 'it's because we're too clever. We shift emotions around and attach feelings to the wrong thing.'

Faye gave her a hard look. 'You mean the wrong men?'

'Yes, but other things too. Like eating as a response to unhappiness when eating should only be the way you respond to hunger.'

'Pete and I were talking about that before you joined us. I think I understand it in theory anyway. I tell you what though, I'm getting myself organised with the Fat Burning Pills. Apart from yesterday, I take two every day and I'm riding my bike as well.'

'It's like wild animals, isn't it?' Mo suddenly said.

'What's that got to do with riding a bike?'

'Animals like deer and tigers take exercise, that's why you never see overweight ones.'

'So animals are in touch with their own blueprints are they?' Faye was teasing her. 'What about your cat then? Remember, you introduced him to me the other night when we went back for a cup of tea after the class? Maybe you should bring him with you and get him to Lighten Up.'

'He's not wild. He's been neutered and he doesn't have to hunt. All he has to do is hang about while I open tins for him. Maybe that's the answer for me, too.'

Faye looked puzzled. 'What?'

'Maybe I need to go out hunting more often.'

The conversation looked like taking a girls' night out sort of turn and I don't like being left out so I decided to join in again. 'The problem for cats is they're pretty limited about what sort of exercise they can take. People have got more interesting options. Why don't you start riding your bike again Mo? Now that Faye and Lisa are both out and about on two wheels, it's time you dusted yours off. You used to ride it everywhere.'

'Well, I did get it out a couple of weeks ago but it's a ten year old racing bike. They're really old fashioned now, and harder to ride as well. Lisa thought it was very un-cool.'

We often do not know when we've eaten enough. So wait for five minutes in between courses and, if you're still hungry, then eat.

'That sounds like Lisa,' said Faye. 'Don't you worry about it Mo. Mine's a shopping bike with a basket on the back and the front. At least you don't have to worry about the older ones being stolen.'

'And you'll both be doing yourself more good than Lisa,' I pointed out. 'You haven't got the gears to get you up hills easily, so it's better exercise. See, there's a positive side...'

Mo interrupted me suddenly. 'I've just had a brilliant idea. Why don't we all do the London to Brighton Bike Ride? It's in June so we've got a couple of months to prepare. We could get T Shirts for everybody and go as a team. What do you think?'

Faye looked horrified. 'I can manage two miles to work and back, but do you know how far it is to Brighton?'

'Fifty something miles if we start at Clapham Common with everybody else.' I knew that because I'd been considering it myself. I thought about the bunch of people we'd just left in the Duke's Head and tried to picture them all in matching T-shirts cycling up Ditchling Beacon. I couldn't quite manage it, but I liked the idea. 'We don't all have to ride bikes. We need some people to drive down with the picnic.'

'I can do that.' Faye looked happier.

'I'll suggest it next Friday. And you get credit for the idea, Mo. Do either of you want a pudding?'

'Do I want a pudding?' Mo looked at the menu again. 'No. I'm definitely full. What's more, I think I've just about done the Food Cake for today. I might be short of a piece of fruit, but that's about it. No wild excesses and I feel full. What more could I want?'

I pointed at the piece of pizza on her plate. 'It's not like you to leave anything.'

'That's because I used to be blissfully ignorant of when I'd eaten enough. Now, thanks to all your bright ideas about laying down your knife and fork and waiting five minutes between courses and concentrating on your food, I'm so bloody self aware it's not true. I really upset my mum last Sunday by not having a second helping at lunch and, what made it worse was Dad suddenly announced he was full as well. He said afterwards he'd never had the courage to do it before. This kind of thing breaks up families.'

I didn't want to pursue that one so I changed the subject. 'Do you want to go back to the Duke's Head?' As soon as I said it, I knew I shouldn't have. Mo's face froze.

Faye stepped into the breach. 'Well, since I've really got to make an effort to be nice to myself and lead a more fun and exciting life, why don't you both take me along to the Comedy Club. You know, that new place that just opened? It's like the Comedy Store only a lot cheaper and concessions are half price. I went there for a hen night last week.'

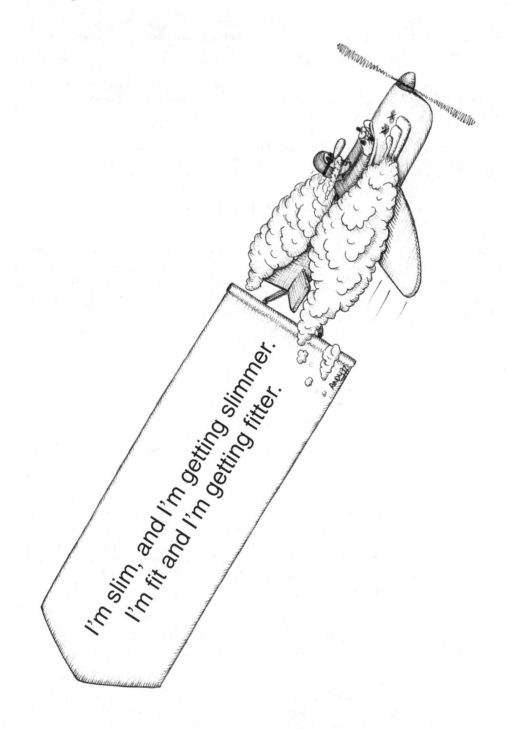

I'm slim, and I'm getting slimmer.
I'm fit and I'm getting fitter.

'How did you manage that?' Mo was temporarily distracted.

'You mean how does someone as old as me know somebody young enough to get married?'

'No, I meant how did you get in on a concession when you're working full time?'

Without any warning Faye grabbed Mo and hugged her. 'There are a few advantages to being over sixty you know. But I'm so pleased you didn't realise.'

We both stared at her. 'You can't be over sixty.'

'Why not? Joan Collins is. So is the Queen.'

The next morning, I'd only had four hours' sleep when the alarm went off. Then I remembered it was Jane's exam and I was covering her Saturday classes. Then I remembered I didn't have either a bike or a car. That ruled out breakfast. I wasn't in good shape when I rushed into the club half an hour later, just fifteen minutes before the first class.

I felt a lot better after a couple of sessions with some good music. Luckily for me the first group was stretching and toning followed by the advanced aerobics so I had time to warm up. I was on my way to the showers when I saw Ben and Lewis at the water dispenser. They waved so I went over. 'How was the karaoke?'

Ben shook his head. 'It was a very strange evening.'

Lewis looked at him very strangely, 'You said it.'

Ben seemed keen to change the subject. 'Where did you and Faye go? And what happened to Mo?'

'We had a pretty lively time in the end.' I told them about the Comedy Club.

'So you had a funny evening in more ways than one,' commented Ben. 'Why not come for a sandwich?'

'Just let me get changed. I'll see you in the café. Or are you going to the pub?'

They looked at each other. 'I'm not sure we'll be allowed back in after last night. We might have to change the Friday night venue to the Slug,' said Lewis, looking meaningfully at Ben.

My heart sank. 'The café then.'

Fifteen minutes later the three of us were seated in a corner of the club coffee bar with enormous prawn and salad sandwiches on walnut bread.

I looked at them. 'Come on. What happened?'

CRAVINGS ARE LIKE WAVES

Don't be wiped out by the urge to eat when you're not hungry

Ride the urge, like surfing a wave. Do something else and the craving to eat will go away

'It was alright until Miriam turned up wearing a very similar outfit to Chris,' explained Lewis.

'It was Donna Karan, according to Lisa,' added Ben, 'and it looked better on Chris. Miriam looked like mutton dressed up as lamb.'

'The point is,' Lewis persisted, 'Chris had been drinking all evening. I asked him where he was going to put all those beers on his food cake and what about his outcomes, just trying to wind him up, you know. But he'd got it into his head that Mo had stood him up and he wasn't listening to anybody. So, Miriam turns up, to find out what we'd all been up to, as usual. And by that time Chris was up on stage doing his Liza Minnelli.'

'Lisa Stansfield,' Ben corrected him.

'I can't tell one from the other. I must be the world's only unmusical Welshman. Anyway, he sees Miriam come in and hauls her up on stage with him. Then he asks everybody to decide who looks best in this dress they were both wearing. Well, everybody stopped talking, you could have heard a pin drop. And you know what Miriam did?'

'No, what?'

'She only grabs the microphone and asks the audience to do a show of hands on whether they think he's male or female! You've got to hand it to Miriam. She knows how to keep calm under fire.'

'So what happened then?'

'Well, everybody thought it was all part of the show and Miriam and Chris carry on trading insults and getting lots of applause until the landlord switches off the mike and announces that if anybody wants that sort of thing they can go to the Vauxhall Tavern but he's not having it in the Duke's Head. And that was it really. The only thing that bothers me is this.'

Ben and I looked at him.

'Why didn't anybody tell me sooner?'

Chapter 9

Transformations And Incantations

I couldn't be bothered to go home straight away so I spent the afternoon in the club addressing my party invitations. The rain was stopping by the time I finished so I walked the long way home and delivered some on the way. Last stop was Mo and Lisa. It was early evening and I wasn't at all sure what mood either of them would be in or even if they would be in.

It must have taken five minutes before I got a reply and I wasn't surprised. I could hear the noise from the far end of the street. Mo eventually answered the door during a brief pause between Pavarotti and Gloria Gaynor.

'What on earth is going on?'

'Lisa's doing her affirmations. It's more like a riot than positive thinking.'

'I'm surprised the neighbours don't complain.' I could feel the floor vibrating slightly. 'What's she doing in there?'

'She skips at the same time. When she first started I had to take the mugs off the shelf.'

I looked up. The dresser was looking pretty bare with no books and no china. 'How long has this been going on?'

'A week.'

'You haven't been tempted to join her then?'

'If I started skipping indoors that would be really bad news for the floor boards.'

'Stop it Mo.'

'Only joking. Anyway, what do you want?'

'I don't always call round because I want something. I've brought your party invitations.'

'You haven't got much choice now we've offered to help. Who else are you inviting?'

'The slimming group plus everybody else I know.'

'Any handsome men?'

'Aren't you going to bring Chris?'

You can have anything you want if you want it with an inner exuberance that erupts through the skin and joins the energy that created the world

Sheila Graham

'Maybe. I haven't forgiven him for last night yet.'

'Ben and Lewis said he drank too much because you didn't show up again.' Suddenly there was silence. Mo sighed deeply and sat down. 'Isn't it just wonderful when she stops?'

Lisa appeared, looking damp and very flushed. She was wearing a silver catsuit. 'Hi Pete, I didn't hear you come in.'

Mo raised her eyes to the ceiling. 'Those affirmations of yours are a health hazard for everybody else. Does it have to be so loud?'

'It works better when it's loud. I haven't found quite the words for me yet so I'm still running variations on "I am slim and fit". When I've got something that's really me, I'll gradually turn down the volume and just do it in my head. Right now, if it's not noisy I'm not convinced.'

'Had you thought of running some affirmations when you take your Fat Burning Pills?' I suggested. 'Fifteen minutes of brisk walking and telling yourself something motivational is less likely to get you evicted. The words are more potent when your body's moving as well.'

Lisa was still bouncing around the kitchen. 'I know. That's why I skip.'

'You never do things by halves, do you?' Mo, in contrast was slumped over the table, motionless. 'The neighbours are going to wonder what's going on.'

'That couple upstairs think we're a pair of witches anyway.'

'Affirmations are kind of like incantations, aren't they?' Mo suggested.

'They really do work better if you put some feeling into them,' I agreed. 'Just sitting in the kitchen going 'I am thin' while you're doing the crossword and stirring your tea is not as effective as it could be. Give it some feeling. Think how footballers behave when they've scored a goal. The elation, the strength, it's physical and emotional all at once.'

'Everybody feels like that after they've scored, don't they?'

'Lisa! Go and wash your mouth out!' I was delighted. Lisa hardly ever made a joke and, for her, it was pretty risqué.

'What I mean is,' said Lisa, pretending to be prim, 'that it's easy to feel that good when you've already succeeded in whatever it is you're trying to do.'

'Ever heard the saying, 'it may never happen?' Well, most great achievements need rehearsing in advance. Unless you do, they will never happen. It's no good just saying the words. Unless you feel the feelings and make the moves, just like you would if you'd actually achieved your goal, you're not creating maximum power for yourself.'

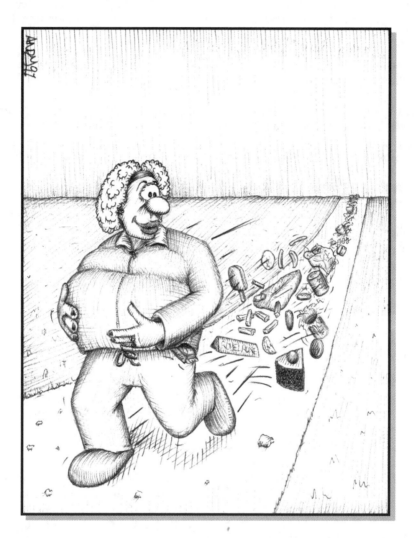

Be Active And Leave The Fat Behind

'You're preaching to the converted,' said Lisa, but Mo looked unconvinced.

'How's everything going for you both, anyway? Can I have some honest feedback please? You promised to be my focus group, remember? What about the Diary, the Food Cake and all the other stuff I've been suggesting?' I sensed personal issues were seething not far below the surface with both of them and I didn't really feel up to it. Losing weight seemed safer than losing relationships or losing control.

Lisa was smug. Unusual for somebody who normally looked like a frightened deer. 'You know I'm really working at it. I'm riding a bike, I'm exercising, I'm doing affirmations and outcomes, I'm even filling up the fat jar. I've got a feeling that this time, it might actually work for me. You may not believe this, but some days I feel quite positive about things.'

'Well,' Mo said, 'you win some and you lose some. I've got a feeling I'm one of the losers – I've gained a couple of pounds.' She was staring blankly at the empty shelves.

'You never told me.' Lisa put a hand on her shoulder.

Mo shrugged her off. 'Why should I? It's none of your business. Anyway, you haven't been around much lately, have you?'

Both Lisa and I were looking at Mo anxiously now. 'Tell me what's not working for you?' I suggested.

'Life's a bit up and down at the moment. We're busy at work and that's good. But, going out with somebody like Chris can be a bit, well, stressful. Exciting but stressful. And the nights when I get home and nobody's in I start feeling low and I eat. End of story.'

'Don't blame me, I can't always be in for dinner.' Lisa was defensive.

'I'm not blaming you. I just feel better if I have something to eat when I'm either watching TV or catching up on the day's paperwork. It feels more complete somehow.'

'What about doing something else instead of eating when you feel fed up?' I suggested.

'Here we go. Displacement activities! I can read you like a book, Pete! In fact, you gave us the book last Friday.' Mo pointed at the list of displacement activities I'd handed out. It was pinned up on the notice board.

'You haven't ticked many.'

'Yes, but we've added a few. Look!'

I got up and walked over to the board. 'That one doesn't count, for a start. Now, tell me what happens, Mo. You walk in through the door. Nobody's in. It's dark. You feel fed up. What do you do?'

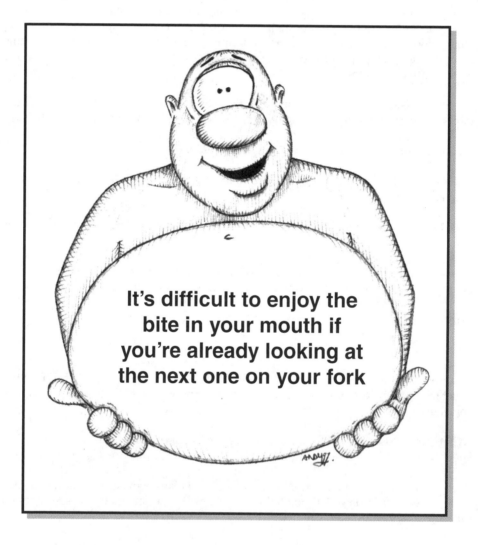

'I feed myself up. And the cat joins me.'

I looked at the cat. He had a habit of sitting on the arm of the chair and I noticed he was starting to overflow on both sides. He looked more like he was draped over the chair arm than sitting on it.

Mo followed my gaze. 'I know what you're thinking. But he doesn't care what he looks like. I wish I didn't care either, then I could just be happy all the time like him.'

'Well, alright then, let's start again. When you get in from work you still feed the cat first. After all, since you took him to the vet he hasn't got anything else much in his life, has he? Then, instead of eating straight away, why not do something else to wind down? You could feed your plants, instead of yourself. Have a chat with them. Lie down on the floor and put one of those meditation tapes on. You've got a whole shelf full. Better still, get yourself a workout video and just do the relaxation exercises on it. Not enough to get sweaty, just enough to revitalise you. Or, how about phoning somebody you haven't spoken to for ages. You're allowed a cup of tea when you do that.'

'I'm not convinced that any of those things will be an adequate substitute for good old comfort eating.'

'They are,' Lisa insisted. 'But you need to get into the habit of them. It may not work the first time, but it's a question of establishing new habits to take the place of old habits that were doing you harm. It's repetition that usually does the trick. Anything can become automatic after a while, it's just that eating is too easy. I do all sorts of things to take my mind off eating and I'm getting quite good at it now.'

Mo gave Lisa a disdainful look. 'I don't want to end up rushing around frenetically like you do, it's not healthy. Anyway, speaking of food, we haven't eaten yet and nobody's asked us out, so we might as well have dinner. What about you, Pete?'

'I'm going to the new James Bond movie. I feel like a couple of hours out of reality. Why don't you come? I remember you telling me, Mo, that Bond women were your role models.'

'OK, but let's eat first. I cooked it already.' Mo pointed at the oven. I'd noticed there was a good smell, but I hadn't made the connection with either of those two cooking real food on a Saturday evening, or any other time.

'My life! You did!' I went right over and patted her on the back. 'You thought, you cooked, you're winning the battle – as Miriam would say.'

'No. Miriam would say you never win the battle and you never stop to congratulate yourself in case you lose ground,' Lisa pointed out. 'Actually, though, I agree with Pete. You know something, Mo, you've been really negative lately but if you just take a look at yourself in the mirror, it must give you some encouragement. You're looking better all the time. I'm going to give you a pat on the back right now, because you're not going to give yourself one. Now, I'll do the rice and the salad. Go and get changed.'

IF YOU'RE NOT HUNGRY...

Walk near trees or a river

Spend a day at the park

Give someone flowers

Buy new underwear

See a movie

Work out at an aerobics class

Go skating

Ride a bike

Picnic

Visit a bird sanctuary

Take up knitting

Decorate a room

Take a day trip

Get a new tape or CD

Begin music lessons

Have a massage

Phone a friend

Organise a game of cards

Book a holiday

See a live football game

Meditate

Learn a language

Volunteer to work for a charity

Wash the leaves on your plants

Share a bath with a friend

Gaze at the stars

Pick fresh fruit

Visit another town

Watch the sunset

Swim at the local pool

Read a book

Window shop

Pet a cat or dog

Send a card

Enrol for a new evening class

Go to a museum

Choose a new plant

Hear some live music

Write a letter

Play tennis

Host a murder evening

Plan a party

Clear out a cupboard

Wash the curtains

Listen to a hypnotic tape

List a week's worth of treats

Join a political party

Draw a picture

'I can go like this,' Mo protested.

'I am not going out with you on a Saturday night looking like that. Have more self respect.'

Mo slunk off to her bedroom and I started setting the table. 'I'm beginning to feel like a permanent fixture in your kitchen.'

'Well, next week we'll be in yours,' said Lisa. 'The party is next Saturday, isn't it? What time do you want us?'

'Are you propositioning Pete?' Mo came back in wearing black jeans with a tight sweater and high-heeled boots.

'No, and what are you doing wearing my jeans?'

'They're not yours. Be reasonable. I couldn't possibly get into your jeans. I liked them on you so I thought I'd try a pair out on me. But then I gained that couple of pounds after I'd bought them, so I never wore them. I just tried them now and, guess what, they don't look too bad.'

'They look wonderful on you. And, hey, that's another displacement activity, buying clothes,' said Lisa.

I thought it was time to make a comment. 'I don't want to be sexist, but I think clothes shopping as a displacement activity works better for women than men. Which is lucky for you, because if watching football is the male equivalent, most men tend to eat while they watch so it defeats the object! Anyway, Mo, since when did you start cooking at home? You always said you wouldn't do that because you had enough of it at work.'

'Well, I don't do much hands-on stuff at work now. I'm mostly on the phone – which is why I've been gaining weight. So I've taken to planning the menus again. I missed it. Also, we're getting a lot more in-house business lunches lately and more and more companies are asking me to put on a 'healthy' option or a vegetarian choice so I'm experimenting with new menus. I test them out back here.'

'Have you tried this one out on the punters yet?'

'No, you're my guinea pigs. It's about my third attempt. It needed more basil and a bit more tomato. I'm relying on the herbs and some garlic to give it flavour. Oh, and a bit of chilli. It's surprising how much you can cut back on the oil and salt when you cook something like this.'

We sat down to eat. When we'd all taken what we wanted, I stood up and moved the serving dishes from the table back to the sink.

'What did you do that for? We might want some more.'

HEALTHY COOKING

Eat plenty of vegetables raw and steamed

Roast vegetables (you don't really need fat)

Trim the fat and the skin from meat

Roast meat and let the fat drain, separate the juice to make gravy

Grill rather than fry

Choose white meat and fish as a protein base

Reduce salt and sugar

Reduce cream and high fat cheese

Reduce the oil you use in cooking and dressings

'It's too easy to keep dipping into the serving dishes if they're right in front of you. It's almost like having it your plate. Oh, and congratulations on leaving some pizza on your plate last night, Mo.'

'Oh, so that's where you went, is it?'

I looked from one to the other. 'You mean you haven't talked about last night?'

'I was afraid to raise the subject,' Lisa said.

Mo looked at her. 'And I was afraid to ask. When I got back to the Duke's Head with Pete and Faye it didn't look like a situation I wanted to be part of.'

Lisa nodded. 'I must admit, I've never seen Chris behave like that, but he is good, isn't he? I don't know what he was like as a chef, but he's a natural on stage. Don't worry Mo, nothing awful happened, we just got thrown out.'

'I heard the story from Ben and Lewis at lunchtime, they were both at the club,' I said.

Mo was looking grimly down at her plate. Lisa caught my eye and put her finger on her lips.

'Well we had a good time, didn't we Mo?' I put a hand on her arm. 'Didn't we?'

'Yes, we did.' She got up. 'Do you want some more of this?'

'Is there enough to freeze?' asked Lisa.

'That's not the point,' I told them. 'If you're really hungry, eat some more. If you get up and leave the table without being satisfied, you'll go on thinking about food and it will get out of proportion.'

Lisa was looking at the leftover casserole. 'And we all know what that means. Popcorn at the cinema.'

'You mean we can't have popcorn?' Mo was smiling again.

'Maybe a small one.'

'No such thing as a small one. There's only large, enormous and ones so big you need to book an extra seat to put it on.'

'I shall take my bottle of water, as usual,' said Lisa.

Mo made a face at her. 'Poser!'

'While you two are worrying about what you might or might not eat an hour from now, I'd like some more of this, please. It's a real winner, Mo.'

Whatever you eat when you're not hungry will be turned into fat

Your body is storing it for later

Just in case you need it

Lisa nodded. Her mouth was full. 'I've still got some hang-ups with food. But I have to admit, from time to time, like tonight, I can really enjoy something again. I haven't done that for years.'

'Mo fetched the cast iron pot back onto the table and I took a spoonful. 'That's plenty, thanks. You've still got enough to freeze.'

'Freezing stuff used to stop me from being tempted to finish it all at once – I couldn't kid myself it was going to waste.'

'Good thinking,' Lisa acknowledged.

'Maybe, but it doesn't seem to be working at the moment – I'm eating the leftovers anyway. These jeans won't be fitting me much longer at this rate.'

I had an idea. 'We could do this bean casserole for the party if you can make large quantities at a time.'

'Aren't you going to stick to bread and cheese and peanuts?'

'I thought I'd do something a bit more substantial than that. After all, I am celebrating a new kitchen.'

Mo got up. 'Seeing as I cooked it, you two can clear away while I go and finish getting ready. I just need five minutes.'

As soon as she'd gone I leaned across to Lisa. 'Why were you trying to shut me up just then?'

'I didn't know just how much Ben and Lewis told you about last night.'

'Just the bit about Miriam and Chris causing a riot.'

'That's all?'

'That's all. Why? What else happened?' I was starting to get worried.

'Well, before Miriam arrived, Ben got up and did a duet with Chris. It was quite amazing.'

'It would be. I'm surprised at Ben. But why should that bother Mo?'

'No reason, I just thought it was odd, that's all.'

'What about you and Ben anyway? Weren't you well on the way to being an item?'

'We've had a couple of pleasant evenings out and I like him very much. But…'

'But what?'

We first make our habits and then our habits make us

John Dryden

'I don't know, maybe he's just shy. It takes longer to get to know people like that.'

I had a feeling she was keeping something back but Mo arrived and, like you always do, we realised we were running out of time to get to the cinema, park the car, buy the tickets and debate the popcorn issue before the programme started.

It was Friday before I saw them again, and then they were both late. I wasn't going to let them get away with sneaking in at the back so I stopped in the middle of my Food Diary review session and asked them. 'What happened to you two?'

'We cooked ourselves a healthy dinner before we came out,' said Lisa, giving me two fingers. 'Give the girls some credit!' shouted Eve, and started off the inevitable round of applause.

'Well, we can see how much in control of their eating patterns Lisa and Mo have become,' I said. 'What about the rest of you? Is anybody else starting to see some changes and feel better about things?'

Ben stood up. 'I have a problem.'

'Come on up here, let's go through it.' "If I can cope with Lewis and his Food Cake I can certainly share a platform with Ben", I thought. 'What's the problem, Ben?'

Ben walked out to the front. He was wearing a track suit again. I'd got used to seeing him in designer cool. In the track suit he looked slightly more like a school teacher than a drug baron. All it needed was a whistle round his neck.

'I can't seem to get rid of this last stone I want to lose.' He said. 'I've got to take the school swimming team to the area gala at the end of the month and I know there's going to be a teacher's race. I haven't gone public in swimming shorts, apart from the beach at home of course, in years. It may not seem important to the rest of you,' he said defensively, 'but I have to keep the pupils' respect. You cannot disguise your belly in swimming shorts. I could be a laughing stock.'

'Alright, Ben. Just tell me exactly what it is that you need to do.'

There was a long pause.

'Well, I need to cut out school dinners and biscuits in the staff room and stick to my packed lunches. I ought to make the time to work out more often too. I know I should do those things, but I keep putting them off.'

'Why? What's the downside?'

'Ah, I get it, it's Pleasure and Pain, is that what you're going to make me do?'

'I can't make you do anything. The question is, can you make yourself do anything?'

Things do not change, we change

Henry David Thoreau

'Alright. If I stop having school dinners, I just eat my sandwiches on my own in the staff room while everybody else is in the canteen. But I enjoy the company. It puts the classes back into perspective when the kids have given you a hard time. And the workouts, well, I do them sometimes. But most nights, I'm just so tired.'

'So, doing things the way you do now, what does that do for you?'

'Well, eating school dinners in the canteen means having a laugh and a gossip with everybody else. Not exercising means I don't have to rush off after school and, again, I suppose, it's hanging out with the others. It's support. Teaching is the sort of job where you need a lot of support.'

'Alright,' I said. 'We've got a clear idea of the pain you're avoiding. Now what will it cost you physically if you don't cut out the jam roly poly and do more of the weights?'

'I will get fatter and fatter. The boys are going to laugh at me. Overweight sports teachers really get some stick. I won't be able to run and keep up with them. That's important.'

'And what else,' I asked, 'will it cost you?'

'Several quid a week in dinners, plus I'm not getting much value out of my club subscription.'

'What will you gain if you make these two changes right away?'

'Oh, I don't know. Self respect, fitness, being able to swim again without being embarrassed, keeping my credibility as a sports teacher, being able to catch the boys when they do something wrong, my brother won't laugh at me when I go home, I won't have to wear braces with a suit, I won't get breathless running upstairs, I won't feel embarrassed when I take my clothes off ...'

There were catcalls from the back row. I raised my hand and stopped them.

'That's a pretty good list, I think you'll agree. Now, Ben, suppose you could just take these actions and make these changes right away? I know you can't, but just think what it would feel like if you could. One way of doing that is to pretend it's already happened. You did the swim. You lost the weight, now retrace the steps you took to get in shape in time for that to happen.'

'If you get into the habit of running through this kind of scenario, it's the start of being in control of your life. If you don't, then life controls you. You already have the ability and the resources you need. You can change your focus and change your behaviour instantly by learning to control pain and pleasure and what you link them to.'

'Let's start from the beginning with this problem. First of all, Ben, just take into account the benefits you get from the dysfunctional behaviour. So, you need company and support at lunchtime. Who wouldn't in your job? Tell me this, could you eat your packed lunch in the canteen? Could you eat it during a free period and just have a cup

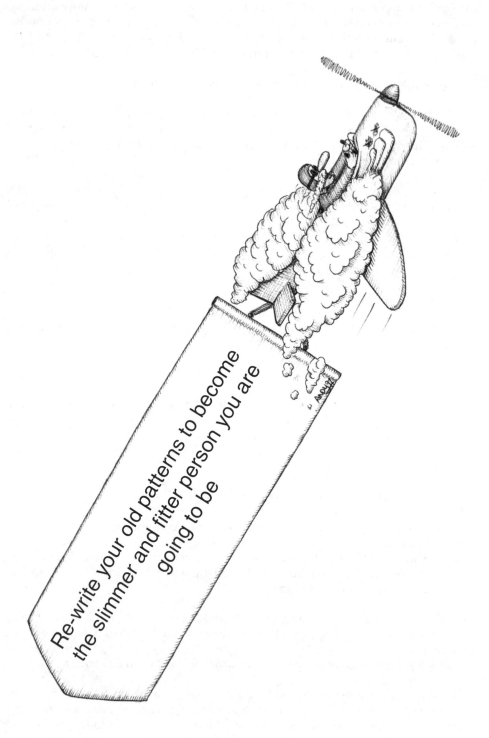

Re-write your old patterns to become the slimmer and fitter person you are going to be

of tea or some fruit in the canteen? How many possibilities are there that would still allow you to socialise with your colleagues and feel like part of the team. Maybe you could start a healthy eating option in the canteen? You may not be the only teacher in the school with concerns about weight and fitness.'

Ben headed back to his seat. 'I'll see. It's not easy to break habits.'

'OK,' I said. 'Anybody else got an issue to raise?'

'I have this problem in the evenings,' said Lisa. 'You know, we were talking about it the other day? You get in from work, you're tired, hungry, nobody to talk to. Nights like that I just lose it. I don't know what to do with myself, there are too many things to do and I don't want to do any of them so I lose it. I nibble, I end up making a snack instead of a proper meal, then I need another snack later, followed by a little something to round off the snacks. Either that or I just get a takeaway and I can never say no to the extra prawn crackers or the special pizza deal where you get free ice-cream and a bottle of coke. The odds are stacked against the single woman.'

'It's worse if you've got a family,' Eve pointed out. 'Single women have it really easy if you ask me. You can eat what you like. When you've got kids you have to get in from work, probably do the shopping on the way, and then cook something everybody likes. And I can tell you it's not cous-cous and fancy bread and posh salads. The only vegetable the younger ones will eat is chips. If it's not deep fried and golden they don't want to know. And the teenagers aren't much better. So what am I supposed to do? Cook for them and make myself a sandwich? I have enough trouble getting them to do their homework and change their socks without trying to educate them about healthy eating as well. I just take the line of least resistance.'

'It's the same with Sean and his dad,' said Faye. 'They don't eat at home much now, but when they did they wanted big, solid meals and I used to be in trouble if there wasn't a pudding. I tell you what though, I had my nieces and nephews to stay for a few days while their mum was in hospital and I got them all colouring in my food cake. In the end I had to take it to work and make a lot more copies so they had one each. They thought it was a real laugh. Kids latch on to something like that sometimes. Mind you, their cakes ended up a funny shape with all the extra bits they added on and I kept having to tell the little one he hadn't got enough green on it.'

'Like Lewis's last week,' Lisa said.

Lewis looked across the room at her. But it wasn't one of his menacing looks. 'Criticising my Food Cake, are you Lisa?' Once again, glances were exchanged.

Eve was still on her theme. 'I'm wondering if your idea might be worth a go, Faye. I hadn't thought of getting the family involved. I've been going to slimming groups that long they just think it's a bit of a laugh at home. Where I come from, it's something mothers do but nobody else bothers. It wouldn't do my husband any harm to lose a couple of stone. I used to be really slim, you know, before I had the children but I just haven't got the time or the money to spend on myself any more. Believe it or not, this is my night out. If you'd told me twenty years ago that my treat for the week would be a slimming club on a Friday evening it would really have upset me.'

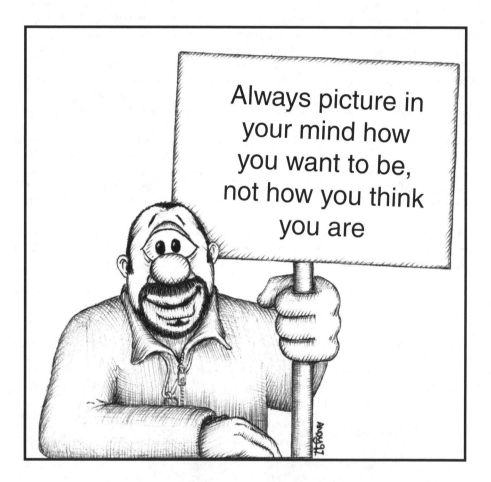

'What does that say about us?' wondered Mo.

I wondered how to help them see that they were all coming at the same problem from different angles. 'Being the size and shape you want to be has wider implications for your lifestyle and your state of mind than most people think. It's about being comfortable and happy in yourself. Or not, as the case may be. That's a pretty important issue whether you're a woman with a family, a rugby player who's past his sell-by date…' Lewis's frown floated on the edge of my vision, like the Cheshire Cat's smile, '…or a business person with an empire to run. Whatever you do, you'll do it better if you're at home in your body and mind. And things like the Food Cake are ways of keeping yourself focused. In fact, there's more to the Food Cake than keeping records. You can use it to take control of what you eat, instead of letting your eating control you.

'From a pink elephant point of view, if you have a graphic image in your mind and on your kitchen wall of what you need to eat, you'll focus on it. Even if you're not doing it consciously, somewhere at the back of your mind you'll know whether you've eaten enough veggies or protein or whatever and you'll be taking steps to make sure you do. It's the first move towards drawing up your own personal eating plan. Not one that somebody else dreamed up for you but one that takes account of what you enjoy eating, the tastes you love, the exercise you take and the way you live.'

After the group I looked in at the aerobics session. Jane was doing it for me again, but I needed an excuse not to get caught up in another Friday night slimming club outing. I was still recovering from last Friday night and I had a party to run the next day. Jane was up front, looking good. Maybe it was just the studying that didn't suit her. At the front of a fitness class she was in her element. She seemed determined to make up for all the times I'd covered for her while she was studying and I was making the most of it.

When the last of the dieters had drifted out, I dashed across the road and sneaked in at the back of St Mark's Hall. Miriam had been on my territory often enough and I thought it was time to pay a return visit. I caught her look of surprise but she didn't miss a beat. When she finished rounding off the session and saying a leisurely goodbye to her group she walked over and sat down in the chair next to me. 'Well, I am honoured,' she said. 'What do you want?'

'Why does everybody assume that I only visit them if I want something? I just want to invite you to my party.' I handed her an invitation. 'I can't promise a low-calorie buffet, but you can bring your own bottled water if you want to keep up the good work.'

Miriam looked at the invitation. 'I think I'm a bit old for this sort of thing.'

'That's not the impression I got from last Friday night.'

She looked alarmed. 'I didn't see you there.'

'I wasn't, but most of my group were. Don't worry, I don't expect you and Chris to put on a repeat performance tomorrow.'

Beans and lentils have very little fat but plenty of protein and complex carbohydrates

Chickpeas

Kidney beans

Lentils

Black eye beans

French beans

Lima beans

Butter beans

You don't even need to wear an anorak, lots of normal people seem to be eating them nowadays. Bread, rice, pasta, cereal and potatoes also contain significant amounts of protein.

'No danger of that. I don't know what came over me. But thanks for the invitation.'

'See you tomorrow.' I headed for home and an early night.

It took me the whole morning to get the music organised and the flat set up for a party. I was just about ready by lunchtime when Lisa and Mo arrived together. 'Nice kitchen. It's wasted on you though. You're hardly ever in. Have you decided on the food? Are we going shopping first?'

I surveyed the kitchen. 'For this many people, it might make more sense to stick to the original plan. Really simple things. Bread, vegetables and some dips.'

'Healthy and cheap as well,' commented Lisa.

Mo waved a piece of paper and a pencil at me. 'Let's make a list. I thought you were going to do my bean casserole. Let's face it, you have a duty to serve something that's good for everybody. You lose credibility otherwise.'

'You're right. The problem with having a lot of things you can pick at is that people do just that without thinking about it. If they've got to actually get a plate and see how much they're eating, there's going to be less of the post-party remorse syndrome. I don't want the slimming group bad mouthing me for the rest of the week. Right. Let's make a list.'

'You know what?' said Lisa, 'Cooking is a real problem area for me. I don't mind doing something like this when we're all working together in the kitchen, having a laugh. But if I'm on my own, I don't bother. "Think Before You Eat" is helpful, but then, when you've decided that what you want is home-made vegetable soup you realise that all you've got is Pot Noodles.'

'That's what I was complaining about and you wouldn't listen,' Mo was obviously annoyed. 'You've been out so much lately that it's not been worth having proper food in the evening.'

'Maybe we could try to eat together more often,' Lisa said, thoughtfully. 'We could make it something simple, early evening, then we can do something else afterwards rather than eating very late and just slobbing out.'

'You can do "Think Before You Cook" as well as "Think Before You Eat",' I suggested.

'That sounds very slimming,' said Mo. 'By the time you've finished thinking you're too tired to pick up a spoon.'

'No, it cuts out all the time-wasting stuff, like starting to eat something you didn't really want, and then finishing it and feeling bad. That kind of thing. But it really does start with planning your shopping and thinking before you cook. That way you know you've got the right things to hand.'

'Say no more,' Mo picked up the paper and pencil again. 'I do it at work, I ought to be able to do it at home.' Between us we worked out a list.

Slow down

Give your new life patterns a chance

Don't say "I haven't got time"

Make time

An hour and a half later, Mo was unpacking the bags, Lisa was making tea and I was panicking. 'It's four o'clock now. People could start arriving at eight thirty and I haven't done anything.'

'Don't worry.' Mo was in her element. 'This is my job, remember? Just stay calm and do as I tell you.' There was a knock at the door. 'That might be Chris, he offered to help.'

I felt annoyed. Then I caught sight of Mo's anxious face as she watched for my reaction. Sanity flowed back. Feeling territorial over a new kitchen – I was ashamed of myself. 'That's great. With two professionals on the case Lisa and me can just KP for you. Why don't you go and let him in?'

Chris stepped through the door carrying a bottle of champagne. 'I thought we could christen the kitchen before everybody else arrives,' he suggested.

Was it my imagination, or did he look a bit wary, a bit less confident than usual? Even so, he seemed determined to be charming and helpful and, best of all, he was dressed like Mo's boyfriend again. To make it even more convincing he hadn't even shaved. He caught my glance. 'Butch or what?' he said and winked at me.

Meanwhile, Mo was getting the ingredients for the casserole lined up. 'Look in that cupboard behind me,' she told Chris. 'The herbs are in there. I couldn't buy all the ones I needed fresh.'

Chris opened the door. 'Hmm, well stocked,' he said approvingly. 'You live by your own rules, I'll give you that.'

I wasn't sure if I was being complimented or patronised but I didn't have time to think about anything for the next few hours. By ten past eight we were as near to ready as we were likely to be. Lisa and Mo disappeared into the bedroom to change and I raised my eyebrows at Chris. 'Aren't you going to put your party frock on?'

'Bitchy,' he said. Then he leaned across the table and lowered his voice. 'How long have you known Ben and Lewis?'

'Oh, I don't really know Lewis. But Ben and me have been friends for years. Why do you want to know?'

'Just curious. Is he going out with Lisa?'

'I'm not sure. They have a common interest in losing weight and they make a pretty stunning couple visually.'

'Being thin and beautiful may not be quite enough,' remarked Chris.

'Who's thin and beautiful?' said Lisa, from the doorway. She was wearing the most amazing black stretch lace dress.

Fat is only a feeling

You have the power to change how you feel

Right here Right now

'Nice,' said Chris. 'What is it? Nicole Farhi?'

'Yes, and thanks, and you're not borrowing it.'

He raised his hands. 'You need to be the genuine article to take risks like that. Where's Mo?'

'Agonising over what to wear. She's brought about six different outfits and she thinks she looks fat in all of them. I told her to just wear those jeans she wore last Saturday but she swears she's put on three pounds this week and she can't do the zip up.'

Chris stood up. 'I believe I'll just go and give her the benefit of my advice.'

Lisa came up to me and put her hands on my shoulders. 'Listen,' she said. 'I have this really good idea.' I felt breathless.

'You look stressed out,' she went on. 'Why don't we all eat before everybody else gets here. You haven't had anything since lunchtime and it's going to be a long night. You never get to eat at your own party.'

I had to laugh.

'What, what's the matter now? What have I said?' Lisa was looking up at me anxiously.

I took her hands off my shoulders. 'Nothing. But that's a brilliant idea. We'll have bean casserole and champagne, NOW!'

The bang from the cork brought Mo and Chris out of the bedroom. He'd obviously worked miracles on her appearance as well as her frame of mind. She was wearing a long, floaty kind of dress with her hair down and her make-up showed signs of borrowed expertise. She accepted a glass of champagne but looked anxiously at the four plates set out on the table.

'I can't possibly eat…'

'You damn well can, and you're going to. For one thing,' said Chris, 'a plate of casserole isn't going to show under that dress, and I don't want you getting drunk and pigging out later on.'

For a minute I thought Mo was going to hit him. Then she shrugged and sat down. 'Maybe I'm getting things back in perspective again,' she said. 'A few weeks ago, if I got upset about something, I'd immediately start feeling fat and I'd just want to crawl away where nobody could see me. Now why on earth should feeling depressed suddenly make you feel fat? I don't know. But it does. Sometimes.'

'That's because you made the association between being fat and feeling bad and you rehearsed it so many times that it became a hard-wired connection.'

Life is short.
Live it up.

Nikita Kruschev

Mo looked up at me, anxiously. 'I suppose so. And once you start thinking like that, the image of yourself as a horrible fat person sort of takes over your brain and you start behaving like a blob as well.'

'But tonight, you didn't do that!' Lisa went over and patted her on the back. 'More strokes for Mo. I want you back the way you used to be. I'm fed up with you being as obsessional as me. One dieter in a household is enough.'

Mo smiled.

Meanwhile, I was thinking about the casserole. 'Being able to change your emotional state without feeling fat is one thing,' I told her, 'but you've changed this as well. It doesn't taste the same as it did when I ate at your flat last weekend. What have you done?'

'I just put different herbs in. It makes a lot of difference. In fact, I put less than last time, and no chilli. So you can taste more of the beans. I've done one pot with chicken in as well and one with tuna. Something for everybody.'

'Do you have any ketchup?' asked Chris, innocently.

When we'd finished shouting at him he said, 'At home, nobody ever ate anything without something on it, you know, relish, or mustard or mayonnaise or whatever. So I used to associate different foods with whatever we covered them in. It wasn't till I started training as a chef that I had to start tasting things by themselves. I mean, fries without ketchup or salt, it was so weird. You never really know what you like and what you don't until you start to get to know what flavours different foods really have. At catering college we were taught that you can disguise badly cooked food if you put enough sauce on it.'

'That's getting back to my blueprint theory,' I reminded him. 'Finding out what you really like. It's about getting back to basics. Besides which, a lot of sauces and dressings are high in fat and sugar and all the rest of it.'

'Leave it out, Pete,' Lisa commented. 'This is a party, remember. If I catch you in a corner with some beautiful person, lecturing her about Fat Burning Pills, there will be trouble!'

Chapter 10

Party On

I want you to know that it definitely didn't work out the way I planned it. Mind you, I'm not sure how I did plan it. I will say though that the food was a great success. I decided to serve it early and get it over with.

The first hour was quiet. Miriam turned up early with a thin, nervous looking man who turned out to be her husband. I noticed that she was trying to stay as far as possible away from Chris who was behaving well and serving the food with Mo. Then, as more people arrived, I got swept up in the party and didn't notice her again until I felt a hand on my shoulder.

'I've got a surprise for you later,' said Miriam. Then she disappeared.

Eve arrived, looking like Elizabeth Taylor before she lost the weight and the hair. Her earrings were amazing. It's a wonder she didn't stretch her earlobes. She was with two beautiful teenage girls who I guessed might be her daughters. I thought, sadly, that she must have looked just like them once. 'Are we allowed to eat what we like tonight, Love?' she asked, 'or is it just crudités and wishful thinking?'

'There's more to a party than the food,' I told her. 'Do you really want to smudge your lipstick? Go and talk to somebody exciting. Introduce these young ladies to Ben and Lewis, you'll make their night.'

'The girls can do their own hunting. I'm here to enjoy myself. My husband's looking after the boys. It won't do him any harm to have a night in for once. I haven't been to a party in ages. And my eldest passed her test today so she's driving. I've got a chauffeur for the first time in my life!'

That was the first thing that made me nervous. Eve had obviously been drinking before she arrived. I decided to change the subject. 'Did Faye come with you?'

'I'm not Faye's bloody keeper. If she's got problems, she'll just have to sort them out herself for once. It's her own fault, she should have thrown the pair of them out years ago. Like Father, like son. And the flat's in her name.'

Fortunately she spotted Chris who, at that moment was waving a French stick, unnecessarily I thought, at Ben. I couldn't hear the joke but from the raucous laughter I could probably have made a good guess.

'Come on girls, you have got to meet Chris. He's the one I told you about.'

Your metabolism is always running higher earlier in the day, so whatever you eat then will be digested more easily than what you eat late in the day.

Daughter Number One giggled. 'He looks, really, you know, normal. I thought he was going to be more like Julian Clary.'

Chris caught the last remark and looked up sharply. He frowned, menacingly, but Eve and her posse were already bearing down on him, shrieking with laughter. I bolted into the kitchen where I found Lisa and Lewis deep in conversation. They didn't notice me come in and I was backing out again when the doorbell rang. They both looked round sharply. Lisa blushed and Lewis looked embarrassed.

When I opened the door, Faye stood on the doorstep looking like a middle-aged Christmas fairy. I'm all in favour of people not dressing their age but I couldn't help feeling that stretch pink shiny jeans was a really bad idea. I felt like wrapping her up in something before presenting her to the party. Her smile was glued on. 'Sorry I'm late. Problems, problems. Still, here I am. And I can smell food. Lead me to it.'

I pushed through the crowd towards the table with Faye slipstreaming me. Mo was serving on her own. Chris, Ben and Eve were out of sight, and dancing had started in the living room. Mo smiled. 'Hello, Faye. Which one would you like?'

'I'll have a bit of everything, please, Sweetheart.'

'You can't do that, it won't mix. Tuna, chicken or veggie?'

'Alright then, I'll start with some of the chicken one. I can always try the others later, can't I?'

'You're going to be dancing with me later,' I told her. That had to be over and above the call of duty I thought.

'It takes several glasses of wine to get me dancing, speaking of which...' she looked around, hopefully.

'I'll get you a drink. Be back in a minute.'

In the kitchen, nothing had changed. 'Are you two glued to the floor or what? What are you waiting for? Have you eaten yet?'

Lisa turned back to Lewis. 'Do you want some food?'

'What about you?'

'No. We all ate before you arrived, so I'm not hungry. Let me get you something.'

'I'm not going to eat on my own.'

'Don't be silly. If you like, you can take your plate over there in the corner and I'll go and dance with somebody till you've finished.'

Lewis looked alarmed. 'Alright. You made your point. I don't mind you watching me eat. You can talk to me.'

ONE BIG MEAL'S NO BIG DEAL

Remember that over-eating isn't important in itself. It's your response that matters.

What's one big meal in the great order of things? The trick is to bounce back. The reaction is more important than the eating itself. Your attitudes are central to your eating both during and after the event.

Over-eating doesn't mean failure

Use it as the opportunity to get feedback so that next time you can do it differently.

That's the secret of success

'Well,' I thought to myself, 'there's a surprise.' When I'd collected the wine I couldn't see Faye anywhere. It's a small flat but people seemed to be disappearing into black holes I didn't know existed. I'd just taken a sip from the glass myself when the music suddenly stopped.

I went into the living room and saw Miriam standing with her hand on the pause button. There were protests from the dancers but, undeterred, she turned up the lights and clapped her hands. When she had everybody's attention, she said, 'I thought I should make a little contribution to this evening, just to show Peter how much I appreciate his refreshing approach to the bitter battle of weight control. I feel we all have something to learn from each other so let's have a round of applause for Mr Cohen.' She looked over my shoulder to the door and nodded at someone behind me, 'You can bring it in now.'

Everybody was clapping and laughing. I looked round, just as Miriam's husband shuffled through the door carrying an enormous cake. It must have been at least two feet across. Or that's how it looked. And it was in the shape of a fat lady in a pink track suit, a bit like one of those Beryl Cook cartoons. She was wearing a beauty queen sash with the words 'Be Your Blueprint' piped on it in icing.

Miriam produced a knife and set about carving it up into large slices which her obedient husband handed round on paper plates. She'd certainly come prepared. People who know me will tell you that I'm not often lost for words, but that night was an exception. I grabbed Miriam by the shoulders. 'What is this about?' I whispered.

She flung her arms round my neck and kissed me on both cheeks. When she was sure we had everybody's attention again she turned back to face her audience, looking sideways at me. 'You mustn't thank me Peter, it was nothing. Just a little gesture from an old hand to a newcomer. Must dash, bye everybody.'

And she was gone. Husband in tow, still clutching a slice of cake. I ran to the door afterwards and watched him take a bite as she dragged him down the path, then they were out of sight. I leaned on the doorpost for a few minutes, then took a deep breath and headed back inside.

The flat seemed to be littered with paper plates and crumbs of the dark, sticky sponge and pink icing. But the music had started again so it seemed like my duty to get the dancing going too.

Somebody grabbed my elbow and I turned around. It was Eve. 'Come and dance, Pete?' I hesitated, she didn't look steady enough on her feet. 'What's the matter? Think I'm past it? That's age-ist, I'll have you know.'

'Pete's going to dance with me? Aren't you?' Faye was at my elbow.

Eve started at her. 'Good grief, Faye, whatever are you wearing?'

'I got ready in a rush. You were supposed to collect me. Remember? I waited for you for ages.'

If you want to
feel good about
yourself and
counter the
negative effects
of stress at the
same time, do
some regular
physical activity.

'I did knock,' said Eve, 'but you didn't answer. All I could hear was your Sean and his dad having a shouting match. I'd got the girls waiting in the car and I decided to leave you to it.' She paused. 'Look, I'm sorry. Fine friend I am. But I've never been any good in that sort of situation. You should take control of it Faye. You don't need those two giving you a hard time.'

'It's alright,' Faye said. 'I understand.' She turned away and slipped through the crowd.

'Oh hell, now I've made it worse.' Eve looked upset. 'I've been such a miserable bag this evening. Parties make me nervous.' She ran after Faye, leaving me feeling distinctly relieved.

Next time I looked at my watch it was half past one and the crowd was thinning out a bit. Faye and Eve had obviously made friends again and they were both dancing happily with a crowd of much younger people but I suddenly realised there were a few faces missing. I went back into the kitchen to get myself some water and see who was still around.

Mo was sitting at the table with her head on her arms. I thought at first she was asleep, but when I touched her on the shoulder she looked up and I could see she'd been crying. I pulled up a chair and put my arm round her.

'What's the matter?'

'I've had four pieces of cake. And I didn't even like it. It tastes synthetic. Even with all the beer I've had I can tell that. I would never serve something that bad. Never.'

'Never mind your professional standards. This is personal. And one lapse isn't the end of the world. Where's Chris? I thought he was going to keep you away from the food.'

She burst into tears again and it took a while to calm her down. Eventually, she was able to speak. 'I can't find him. He went out to the kitchen hours ago when I was still serving the food. And he never came back.'

'Come and dance with me?'

'It's too late for that. You really don't understand, do you? It's over.'

'What's over?'

'Chris and me. It hasn't been right for a few weeks. It's over and so is my attempt to compete with Lisa. I'm admitting defeat. I'm podgy and disgusting. I don't know why I ever thought that someone like Chris would stay very long with someone like me. I want to go home.'

The quality of your life depends on the questions you ask yourself

What you focus on is what you get. Try asking more empowering questions like:

"What can I do today that will move me forward.

"How can I become slimmer right now"?

or

"What can I do today that will keep me going on the road to becoming slimmer?"

I looked around but I couldn't see anyone Mo knew. 'Where's Lisa?'

'I don't know and I don't care. I haven't seen her since the beginning of the evening.'

'Well,' I told her, 'you've got two choices. I can call you a taxi or you can sleep in the living room here.'

'Oh, great, I can sleep in the remains of the chocolate cake. I suppose you think I can just eat the rest of it and save you having to clear it up in the morning. Call me a taxi, please. I've had as much as I can cope with.'

Next morning was pure hell. By lunchtime I was still scraping icing off the wall. I was relieved when the doorbell rang. Any distraction was welcome.

Lisa was on the doorstep. 'I thought you might need a hand. Look!' She opened her shoulder bag. It was full of rubber gloves and cleaning materials. 'Men never have enough stuff to clean a kitchen properly. How far have you got?' She paused at the entrance to the kitchen. 'Oh. Not far.'

With two of us on the case it seemed to go more than twice as fast. 'You know,' said Lisa, 'last night was the first time in ages that I didn't seriously pig-out at a party. I had a piece of that disgusting cake – which I didn't mean to – but that was all.'

'That was a lapse,' I told her. 'You're bound to have the odd lapse, but it doesn't matter. Put it behind you and get on with life.'

'Yes, but normally I would have upset myself by having the cake, then I'd have kept thinking about it – and I don't have to tell you what happens when you keep thinking about something …'

'But last night was different for you.'

'It certainly was.' She stopped with a scouring pad in one hand and a rice pan in the other.

'I'm talking about chocolate cake,' I reminded her.

'Oh, yes. Right. Anyway, I just had the one piece. I haven't had anything sweet like that since I gave up the Kit Kats after work. I must admit, it hit the spot. Just like it used to, but at the same time, it didn't taste very good. And then I stopped and I looked down at myself – remember that dress I was wearing?'

'That dress is unforgettable. But what's it got to do with the cake?'

'Well, the Food Diary and all that other self awareness stuff you keep banging on about seems to be sneaking up on me. I keep stopping and running these little "how do I feel about this?" tests on myself. I did one then. It's just momentary when you get into the habit of it. I was thinking 'OK, Lisa, you got the sugar high, but what is all this

LISTEN TO YOUR BODY

Create A Picture Of Health

You have all the tools you need to live
a healthy life

So, loosen up a little, be flexible with
yourself. Listen to what your body is
telling you and act accordingly

Lighten up and lighten the load

mock-chocolate sludge going to do to your body? And if you get back into the habit of eating this crap then are you going to go on looking as good as you look now?' And last night I did look good and I felt good too. Well, by that time I could virtually feel the cholesterol accumulating in my arteries and the fat cells getting all plump and wobbly. It was not actually that difficult to turn away from temptation. The teachers at school always said I had too much imagination, but I think I may have found a good use for it at last.' She bent over the pan and scrubbed vigorously. I noticed she was smiling.

'Brilliant.' I patted her on the back. 'Give yourself some credit. You've learned something incredibly important and we aren't even due to cover it in the group till next Friday. I'm going to be talking about how to tell the difference between a lapse, a relapse and a total collapse.'

'So, I just had a little lapse. Nothing to worry about. But what's a relapse?'

'A relapse is stringing a bunch of lapses together. Like, if you'd had a couple more pieces of cake and then, this morning, you'd have felt bad about it and decided the weekend was a write-off so you'd go out, eat a load of croissants and wash them down with a couple of large cappuccinos. Then, Monday morning, you'd pull yourself together and get back to the clean living until you fell into temptation again in the next weak moment.'

'Sounds familiar.' Lisa continued scrubbing.

'Lapses and Relapses are nothing to worry about. They are just behaviour patterns. You can change them. Collapses are more serious because they are based on beliefs, not behaviour.'

'Well, the difference may be obvious to you, but it's not obvious to me.'

'Collapse only happens when you start believing your old negative beliefs about yourself again. When you start to think you're always going to be fighting the battle against overweight, you get battle weary. When you start carrying around that permanent image of yourself being plain and plump, it's easy to just behave like a plain, plump person, eat like a plain plump person, slob about like a plain, plump person. But you felt good about yourself last night. You felt like a beautiful, slim, loveable woman and women like that don't need chemicals at a party. It would have taken more than one slice of cake to knock you off course, wouldn't it?'

'Yes, you're right. It's a different feeling, a different belief, a different self image. I thought it was something that just happened by itself. But when I look back over the past couple of months, I suppose I can take some credit. I've been working at it.'

'Remember Lisa, weeks ago, when we went for that walk, one of the things you said you believed you had going for you was your determination. You never give up so you did all the daft things I suggested even though you didn't believe them at first. You stuck at it, and now you do believe some good things about yourself, everything's getting easier, right?'

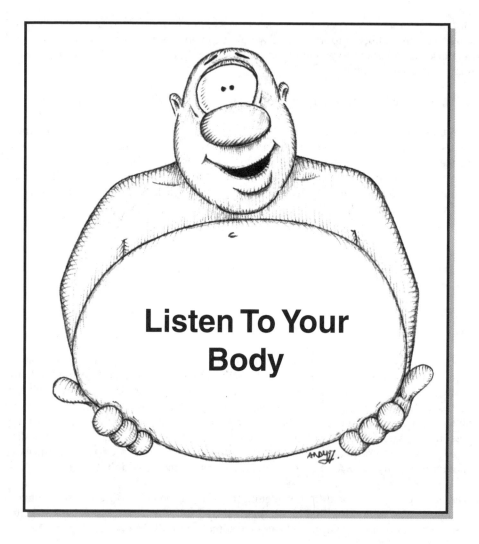

'She looked at me and smiled. Yes, yes and yes. I suppose. But you know this stuff about lapses? I've been destroyed by lapses in the past, I've stuck to a diet for weeks and then it's all fallen apart in the course of a weekend. How can I be sure it won't happen to me again? I'm afraid of that. I can't bear to lose what I've got now.'

'Your state of mind is much more important than your behaviour and you've already made some big changes in your state of mind. If you keep those changes, continue to do your affirmations, set your outcomes, and "Think Before You Eat", a collapse becomes increasingly unlikely. It's the mind-work that matters, not a few thousand calories here and there. That's the difference between a relapse and a complete collapse. And you said yourself that some of those little mental exercises are automatic for you now. You're re-wiring your circuits. By the way, changing the subject for a minute, did you talk to Mo this morning? I was really worried about her last night. She'd eaten too much and she was crying in the kitchen and talking about giving up.'

There was a pause. Lisa avoided my eyes. 'She'd already gone to bed when I got in and she was still asleep when I looked in on her this morning.'

'Wait a minute, she left the party after you.'

Lisa coughed. 'Lewis and I went for a quiet drink, Pete. Sorry I didn't stay till the end, but it was so noisy and we seemed to have a lot to talk about.'

After a second I realised I was staring at her with my mouth open. I pulled myself together. 'You and Lewis?'

She was defensive now. 'Sure, he seems a bit aggressive but, when you get to know him, he's really straightforward and nice.'

I wasn't sure about the nice. 'What about Ben?'

'I don't know,' Lisa said, irritably, 'I only saw him for a few minutes right at the beginning. He's avoiding me since we…, anyway, never mind Ben, you've got me worrying about Mo as well now. I'll do a bit more here then I'll head for home and see how she is.' She paused. 'Do you think she's collapsed?'

After Lisa had gone, I cooked myself a meal and finished off the clearing up. Then I had a blissfully early night. On the way home from work next day I called in to see Mo. Somehow I didn't expect Lisa to be there and I was right. It was past eight by the time I arrived but Mo had only just got in.

'You're not usually this late,' I said.

'Work's about the only thing that's going right at the moment. Come on in.' She unlocked the door.

I think the one lesson I have learned is that there is no substitute for paying attention

Diana Sawyer

'I was worried about you after the party,' I told her.

'Thanks. I'm OK. Just going through a bit of a bad patch, that's all.'

I sat down and watched as she took off her coat and switched on the kettle. 'What actually went wrong at the party?'

'What didn't? When I thought everybody had finished eating, I was clearing up some plates when Faye came up and was nice to me.'

'What was wrong with that?'

'I was feeling fed up. Everybody else was having such a good time. Faye got us both another plate of food each and we sat down together in the corner. She said she fancied some more and she felt guilty about eating on her own. I had it to keep her company really. Then she went to get drinks for us and, while she was gone, Miriam came and sat down with me. She said how pretty my dress was and then she went, "you can eat as much as you like in a dress like that. Nobody's going to notice, are they?" and after that I just kept hearing her voice saying "eat as much as you like, nobody's going to notice". It was, like she was really saying "nobody's going to care". That's how I felt. Then she brought on that cake and the rest, as they say, is history.'

'Honestly, Mo, you've got to remember that eating too much occasionally doesn't really matter. It's how you cope with it that makes the difference. So you ate too much. It's over now. Why not just get back to your own personalised Food Cake?'

As she took down the mugs, she glanced back over her shoulder at me. 'I did all the right things on Saturday to begin with, didn't I? We ate beforehand so we weren't starving. There weren't any little bits to keep picking at and I didn't mean to get a plate and go and have another serving of that casserole, never mind the cake. One reason I offered to help was so I could be serving rather than eating. It's a good way of getting to meet people as well. It just went out of control.'

'What did you do all day Sunday? I called you after Lisa left, but you didn't answer.'

'I went home for lunch. I thought it might cheer me up a bit. But it was like an action replay. My auntie was there and both grannies, and they seem to think that the answer to all life's problems is a cup of tea and another helping of pudding. I told them I was still full from the night before and Mum went all huffy. She said there wasn't much point in her spending all morning cooking Sunday lunch if nobody was going to eat it. Then Dad took me on one side and told me not to cause trouble because we were still in the dog house for not having second helpings last week. So I just gave in and went with the flow. I stayed for tea as well. The big logistics problem in our house on a Sunday is getting the lunch things washed up in time to start putting the tea things out for half past five.'

'You have to be firm, Mo. This is your life, your body and your wellbeing you're dealing with.'

'I know that. In theory.' She passed me a cup of tea and sat down.

LEARNING THINGS YOU NEVER KNEW YOU NEVER KNEW

Controlling your weight isn't really learning something new. It's about re-learning the knowledge your body was born with but which your conscious mind may have decided, for lots of social reasons, to over-ride.

'In situations like family lunches and parties, you have to plan in advance. If you know you're going to be in a difficult situation food-wise, prepare yourself. Then you won't get caught off balance and you'll be able to say that you are fine and that the best way they can help you is by ignoring your diet and not pushing food at you.'

'It's hard when they're trying to show they love you and you need all the love you can get.'

'Love yourself first. You're not doing too well with that at the moment, are you?'

'Look, Pete, I don't want to be rude or anything, but I've got my VAT returns to do. Would you mind if I don't ask you to stay for dinner?'

'I'll cook for you and you can make a start on the VAT forms while I'm doing it,' I suggested.

'No, really … actually, I ate on the way home. That's why I'm late. And I'm not going to tell you what I ate. I know you mean well, but just go.'

I hadn't even finished my tea, but I know when I'm being thrown out so I got up and grabbed my hat. 'See you Friday,' and left.

By the time Friday night arrived, I was quite nervous. So far I'd only seen Mo and Lisa since the party and, so far the reviews had been 50% for and 50% against.

Faye and Eve arrived together. They came straight up and thanked me for the party. 'What was Miriam about with that cake?' asked Eve.

'Malicious cow,' said Faye. 'I may have had a couple of drinks on Saturday night, but I know sabotage when I see it. She was just trying to prove a point.'

'What point?'

'Why don't you ask her?'

I looked around. Miriam was standing in the doorway. She looked embarrassed.

'Well?' I looked at her enquiringly.

'Just came to say thank you, Peter. Lovely party. We both enjoyed it. Kevin doesn't get out much …'

'I'm not surprised,' muttered Eve. Miriam looked at her sharply.

'Explain the cake to me,' I said. 'Assume that I'm really stupid and I didn't get the message first time around.'

TREAT YOUR BODY WITH RESPECT

Listen to your body

Love it

Give yourself positive messages every day

Feed your body with nutritious 'living' food and cleanse it with pure water

Exercise it

Rest it

Enjoy it

Miriam took a deep breath. 'Well, it's called the piranha principle. If you throw a piece of raw meat into a piranha pool the result is feeding frenzy. It's their nature. Their blueprint if you like. They smell blood and they just lose control. Did you notice the reaction when Kevin started handing round that cake? Your diet group couldn't stuff it down themselves fast enough. It's because that's their blueprint. Give them sugar and fat with a bit of chocolate thrown in and whatever nonsense you've tried to teach them about listening to their bodies is out of the window. Because they are listening to their bodies. That combination is delicious. I know it. You know it. It's an instant fix of happy energy. If they'd been a bunch of junkies I could have handed out cocaine. The only thing that works with weight loss is constantly reminding people that they're fighting a battle for life and helping them to fight it.'

'Listen, Miriam, there was a time when I would have agreed with you.' Faye stepped forward. 'But, you know why I don't come to your groups any more? Because it's a hiding to nothing, that's why. I lost weight, then I put it on again, plus a bit more. It was the same story over and over and over again. The only long term changes were that every time I dieted I ended up a pound or so heavier in the long run and I was getting steadily more depressed about it. You were fighting the battle for me, so of course, I was never going to win it. I can't be you.

Since I've been doing the Lighten Up course, I've lost several pounds. It's not dramatic but I feel like a new woman. And I'm starting to believe that I can really be whatever weight I want to be, I just have to get a life first.'

'Forgive me for raising this, Faye, but you didn't look to be on top form last Saturday,' Miriam pointed out.

'You left too early, Miriam. I haven't enjoyed a party so much for ages. It's ages since anybody asked me to one. In fact, the reason I had such a good time was thanks to you.'

'What do you mean?' Eve and Miriam both looked at her.

'I headed for the food as soon as I arrived. I always do that. It gives me something to do so I don't stand around feeling shy and awkward. I even spotted Mo looking a bit down and I got her to eat with me when I went back the second time. I feel bad about that too. I mean, not only was I eating for the wrong reasons, I was pushing someone else into doing the same thing. Poor girl, I must speak to her later. Anyway, Miriam, when you turned up with the cake, I suddenly realised what a fool I was being. Apart from the fact that it was obviously meant to be me, although I can't imagine how you knew I'd be wearing pink, I suddenly realised how stupid it all was.'

She had everybody's attention now.

'I can sit at home and eat cheap cake whenever I like. I watched everybody else digging in and I thought, 'ten years ago, twenty years ago, that would have been me.' You know what I did? I went and introduced myself to a few people. I shared a few jokes, had a laugh or two. When you're older, you can get away with it. You're not so self conscious. Then Eve came in and we started dancing. By the time I realised how tired I was there wasn't any food left anyway.'

THINKING LIKE EDISON

Edison was given the finance to make an electric light bulb, an idea which had been the despair of inventors for 50 years. It took him 14 months of trial and error to find a suitable filament and he got it wrong hundreds of times before he got it right. But every time he tried an unsuitable material he merely took the view that he had simply eliminated another possibility and was one step closer to finding a permanent solution to the challenge.

'Well, on that inspirational note I'm afraid I have to leave you.' Miriam turned on her pointed heels and left.

I turned to Faye. 'Are you really shy? You're the last person I would have expected to have trouble with parties?'

'Everybody is.'

I looked round.

Chris had just walked through the door. He came right up to Faye and put his arm round her. 'Everybody gets nervous in social situations. Big parties are just the pits for everybody. So what does any sane person do? They do something familiar and comforting. They eat. The next most stressful situation is the family party. That's a different kind of pressure because everybody's known you since before you had any style. You turn up and everybody's putting all these expectations on you. "You're so tall, you remind me of your father, "Why don't you get a proper job?", "We don't see much of you these days." All of that stuff. And so you eat to make them think you're normal. "Oh, don't ask me about work, but isn't this cheesecake delicious?" Anyway, Faye's obviously put all that behind her, haven't you, Darling. There's only one thing I'll say to you, though,' he gave her a hug, 'next time there's a party I'm going to come right round to your house and be your fashion advisor.'

Faye slapped him playfully, but she was laughing. 'You can have those pink jeans for your act if you like,' she said. 'I've got a feeling I won't be wearing them again.'

'They won't fit you for much longer,' Chris told her. 'they'll be much too baggy.' He turned to Eve. 'And as for you – I'm surprised you can look me in the face after Saturday. A fine example to your children you are.'

Eve blushed. 'You should be able to cope with a bit of teasing. Especially if you go around looking like Danny la Rue half the time. You must be used to it by now.'

'Danny la Rue!' Chris looked absolutely thunderous.

'Eve means Julian Clary of course, don't you, Sweetheart? You've got to try and keep up,' said Faye.

'I like Julian Clary,' said Ben. 'I saw him do a live show once. Come on, let's get started then we can go for a beer.' He and Chris took their seats and looked at me pointedly.

When everybody had settled in I decided to lay the party ghost. 'It was nice to see so many of you last Saturday. I hope you all enjoyed it.'

A buzz went around and Eve said, 'Was the party part of the course? If it was an exam, did we pass or fail?'

YOU CAN DO IT

It's up to you. You have the resources, and the knowledge, to make the difference you want to make to your life. The only person who can make you slimmer is you. There's no diet or magic formula that will transform your life.

The responsibility is yours

'It's not a question of passing or failing. I know that some of you felt they had a bit of a lapse in terms of their eating schedules, particularly when Miriam arrived with the chocolate cake. I also know that some of you didn't get washed off course by the avalanche of sugar and fat and that you found other ways of coping with social situations than just eating. It's easier to talk and listen if you're not stuffing your face with food. In fact, you make yourself very popular by being more sensitive to other people's social needs than if you're concentrating on running away from your own social inadequacy.'

'Harsh words,' said Chris.

Ben was nodding. 'Rings bells though. Most people are hopeless at parties. I used to think it was just me. But it isn't.'

'Yes,' Lisa called from the side. 'The main thing to remember is that it's not the lapse that matters, it's your response to it that makes the difference. It only becomes a total collapse when you stop believing that you can be slim. Right, Pete?'

I nodded. 'Give me some examples of things you believe in.'

'Here we go. He's off, we'll all be chanting again in a minute,' said Lewis.

Lisa gave him a look from across the room and he shrugged at her and grinned. I noticed that Mo hadn't turned up.

'Alright,' Chris said, 'I'll start the ball rolling. I believe I'm half a stone overweight.'

'I'm three stone over,' said Faye.

Lisa protested. 'What sort of belief is that to have about yourselves? If you believe you're overweight, you're never going to be any different, are you? Every time somebody offers you a Danish pastry you'll fall for it. Because you don't really believe you'll ever change. The difference happened for me when I started to believe I was going to be slimmer and I focused on the future. I'd been doing the affirmations but I wasn't taking them seriously at first.'

'The neighbours were though, from what I heard,' said Ben.

Lisa looked at him thoughtfully for a moment. 'I'd forgotten you were around at the high decibel phase, Ben. Anyway, like I was saying, one minute my affirmations were just words – "I am slim and fit and full of energy" and then gradually they started to feel quite reasonable. One day I suddenly found myself thinking, "Yeah, I can believe that", and from then onwards it was a lot easier to say "no, thank you" when somebody offered me something my body didn't need.'

Silence followed this moving testimonial to the power of self belief.

SMILE

Every time you smile, you relax all the major facial muscles and you get to feel good as well

Try it more often

'The point about beliefs,' I told them, 'is that they have to be supported by something or they won't stand up to pressure. If you're going to adopt a new and life enhancing belief about yourself, you've got to make sure you've got plenty of reference points to back it up.'

'Like what?' asked Ben.

'Like "I'm doing the Lighten Up programme",' I suggested.

'I'm thinking before I eat,' said Chris.

'I'm riding my bike to work,' suggested Lisa.

Faye put up her hand. 'I'm too old to wear shiny pink jeans.'

Eve put an arm round her. 'No, Faye, love, what you mean is, "I'm too classy to wear shiny pink jeans".'

Chapter 11

Failure And Feedback

I was worried about Mo, but I didn't a get chance to talk to anybody about her after the Lighten Up group. I was running the aerobic class immediately afterwards because Jane had taken an Easter holiday.

I didn't expect any of the Lighten Up punters, but Lisa sneaked in during the warm-up. She didn't seem to be working as hard as usual and, at the end, I grabbed her before she headed for the changing rooms. As soon as I got closer I could see the problem. Her eyes were red, her skin was blotchy and she looked ill.

'What's the matter?'

'I started a cold last night. I think it's flu. I'm aching all over.'

'Why didn't you go straight home after work and get an early night?'

'Well, this exercise programme is going so well, I didn't want to miss one. Sometimes you can just shake something off.'

'Remember the blueprint? You should have been listening to your body, giving yourself a bit more respect.'

'I'm afraid that if there's a blip in the routine, I'm going to lose it altogether, like I did before.'

'Lisa, you're on the verge of pushing yourself too hard again. You're still on the knife edge between success and failure. It's not like that. It's a gradual process of getting to know yourself and letting your body settle down into an exercise and eating routine that's right for you. If you wait while I close down here, I'll run you home. My car was fixed yesterday.'

'That would be great. Just give me ten minutes to change.'

I was sure I could be ready faster than Lisa, but I'd under-estimated the difference it would make if she wasn't bothering with the make-up and hairstyling routine. She was already waiting for me when I got to the entrance and she was looking worse than ever. When we arrived at the flat I parked the car and followed her in. Mo was huddled over a pile of books and printouts, with a glass of wine and a box of matzos beside her. 'Where were you tonight?' I asked her.

She didn't look up and she didn't answer the question. 'Was Chris there?'

'Yes.'

WHEN PEOPLE TRY TO MAKE YOU EAT

Sometimes people will try to make you eat and you can have fun tailoring your avoidance strategy to their motivation. Just ask yourself what they really mean when they say "try one of these – they're yummy."

"I'm out to sabotage you"

"It's the only way I know to show I love you"

"It's the only way I know to ask you if you love me"

"It's the only way I know to be sociable"

"I'm miserable. I'm going to overeat and I want company"

'I suppose he went to the pub afterwards?'

'I don't know. I had a class.'

Mo got up slowly and went over to the kettle. 'I'll make you some hot lemon, Lisa. I told you not to go.' Lisa patted her and disappeared to her room.

'What's the matter, Mo? Is it just about Chris?'

'I don't know. Everything seems to be connected with everything else, doesn't it? You feel fat, you get rejected, you feel fatter. And uglier. At least all the stress has coincided with the end of the tax year so I've got nothing to distract me from getting the books in order.'

'What about your Fat Jar? What about Thinking Before You Eat? What about your Affirmations and your Outcomes?'

'I can't seem to focus on them at the moment. It's no good me sitting on the train every day saying "I am losing weight and becoming more attractive"' when I don't believe it, is there? I'm not eating that much because I'm never really hungry, but the weight's creeping back on.'

'At least you're still logging on to your Hunger Scale then.'

'Not consciously. It's automatic now – like a lot of those things you made us think about. Even when I'm going through a phase like this, I can't completely escape into all my old bad habits.'

'Did you get around to drawing up your Personal Eating Plan?' I asked her.

'No, I was using the Food Cake, but the last few days I've just been grabbing a snack here and there.'

'You know what's happening then, don't you? You're body's slowed down your metabolism because it doesn't know where the next meal's coming from and because you're not exercising. Those snacks are probably crisps and biscuits and doughnuts and stuff – the good old sugar and fat combinations – so you're playing havoc with your digestion. You're getting the sugar highs, then the munchies. You don't know how you feel any more.'

'Don't lecture me, Pete. I can't take it. I'll try again after Easter. I might do a real serious diet and workout combination for a couple of weeks and then, when the weight starts to shift, I'll go back to your organic system again.'

Lisa put her head round the door. 'I'm going to bed. Goodnight everybody.'

'Before you disappear, admit to me that you were mad to do the aerobics.'

The one word you'll need is 'NO'

Bette Davis to Robin Williams

'Pete, I've already apologised to myself. I've learned my lesson. What do you call it? Not failure but feedback? Oh, and thanks for the lift.'

She disappeared and Mo sat down again in front of her papers.

'Listen, Mo, you're stressed and unhappy, I can tell. That's a bad combination and what you're doing isn't going to help.'

'Work takes my mind off things.'

'Yes, but you need to relax. Relaxation is the only cure for stress. Overworking, bad eating and under-exercising will only make it worse.'

'How can I relax when I'm stressed and unhappy? It's a contradiction in terms.'

'Do you want to lose that weight you think you just put back on?'

'Of course I do. I just don't believe it's possible when I'm going through a bad patch in my life. You can only stick with a weight control program when you're reasonably happy. When you're feeling down you need chips and chocolate and wine and you don't have the energy for gratuitous exercise.'

'So, if something goes wrong in your life, you're bound to eat and drink too much and gain weight? You really believe that?'

'Why shouldn't I believe it? It's always been true for me in the past.'

'You're compounding the pain. When you stop being depressed about whatever it was that triggered off your downward spiral, you'll be left with the fallout. Long after you've come to terms with the original pain, you'll be stuck with an extra half stone and a load of bad habits.'

'OK, so what can I do?'

'You can start knocking the legs out from under that belief straight away. And when it falls over, you can start believing more positive things again.'

'How?'

'Well, apart from the fact that it's always happened before, how do you know you'll always get fat when you're unhappy?'

'I snack on all the wrong things, just for comfort, I feel too lethargic to exercise, I can't be bothered to go anywhere and do anything I don't have to …'

'But now, you have displacement activities you can do instead of nibbling, you've got into the habit of exercising so it's not a big deal like it used to be, you've got people who expect you to go out and have fun with them, you've got me nagging you for free, you've got a Food Cake, you've got a lot more options than you ever had before!'

THE FOOD AVOIDER'S PHRASEBOOK

It *looks* wonderful but …

I can't make up my mind now, I'm going to come back later …

I'm just going to get a drink / dance with / talk to / catch up on …

I'm just taking a tiny bit to start with because I know I'll be nibbling all night.

Please let me have the recipe for this, let me find a pen and paper …

I can't wait to try it, but first I just have to go to the loo / fix my face.

Have I told you about … (it had better be a good story).

I'd love some more salad (lettuce fills a plate and you can push it around for ages).

It smells so good – tell me what everything is and then leave me to decide.

I'm taking food allergy tests at the moment and this is my cucumber week

I must just go and tell my husband / boyfriend / minder / walker that dinner's served.

I had to go and visit my Granny on the way here and she's been feeding me fruitcake.

I had food poisoning yesterday but I'm alright now as long as I don't eat anything.

Just then the doorbell rang. I was already standing up so I went and opened it. Ben and Chris were on the doorstep with a carrier bag from the off-licence on the corner. I was just about to let them in when I realised that Mo had followed me up the stairs and was right behind me.

'We missed you and Lisa at the pub,' said Chris, 'so we thought we'd bring the pub to you.'

Mo pushed past me and confronted them. 'We're both busy. Lisa's having flu at the moment and I'm about to try a new displacement activity. I'm going to have a bath in green jelly. It should be a good substitute for you. Slimy bastard.' She pushed past me and slammed the door in their faces. Then she stood, just staring at the back of it. 'I cannot believe they actually came here together!'

'I take it that now isn't a good time to discuss relaxation techniques then?' I asked her.

'Afraid not. I've had as much help and advice as I can cope with for one evening. If I'm going to be miserable, I might as well enjoy it. I'm going to have a good wallow in self pity. It's a great relaxation technique, Pete, you should try it.'

'See you next Friday then. It's the last Lighten Up group.'

'Maybe. Bye.' Mo disappeared down the stairs.

That Friday I had lunch with Jane again. She was looking good after her holiday, and I noticed she was back to the shiny lycra without the baggy T-shirts.

'Guess what?' she handed me my baked potato. 'I passed the exam.'

'Congratulations!'

'You remember last time we had lunch? You were lecturing me about rushing my food. Well, during that two months when I was studying I gained ten pounds. That's never happened to me before, even when I was doing GCSEs. It made me a bit more sympathetic to all the people I see who are always banging on about their weight. I thought I might come along to your Lighten Up course and see how it's done. I got back on form quite quickly, but I can see now how difficult it must be for people who aren't fit to start with. And there's something else I wanted to ask you. I saw you doing relaxation techniques in a class the other day, and I thought, "I could do with some of those". Then, next time I'm studying, maybe I won't get so wound up about it and resort to the Yorkie bars.'

'Surely you learned all about relaxation techniques in college?'

'It was never my strong point. I've always been better at doing things than not doing things. That's why I don't like sitting still and reading. I have to do something else at the same time, like eat! While I was studying I couldn't even sleep properly, then I'd fall asleep over my books.'

SAVING YOURSELF

If you aren't assertive, don't be caught out. Rehearse answers for eating-pressure situations.

Eat beforehand.

Eat only special foods – decide to go for the salad or sandwiches not crisps and dips.

Eat slowly. Start last and make it last.

Talk to other people about the food, praise the taste and style and presentation.

Sit down to eat. Then you'll be more aware of starting and finishing.

Take what you want from the buffet table and eat it somewhere else.

Just think, this is the only place and time when you can **talk** to this particular group of people but you can eat at home anytime. Somebody in this room might change your life - with an idea, a job opportunity, a personal revelation or a new love affair. Eating is something you can do by yourself. Anytime.

Dance a lot. If nobody else is dancing, get them started.

Offer to help in order to stay occupied.

*Think how you will feel when you leave knowing that you **haven't** over-eaten.*

I went over to the drawer for some forks and handed her one. 'The thing about relaxation techniques is that you have to find the ones that suit you best and practice them. Exercise is a good form of relaxation for somebody like you. If you build up a lifestyle that includes a lot of physical activity, you can't stop, just like that and sit at a desk for two months. You needed to take time out to work out every day. You would have been less tired because you'd have got rid of your excess tension. Whatever relaxes you reduces the effect of the stress hormones you're producing. It's bound to improve your sleep pattern as well, because you'll be able to shut off and relax.'

Jane nodded. 'But there are two different versions of me. One is the successful fitness instructor. When I'm in that mode I don't suffer from stress, or insomnia or gaining weight. That version of me works really well. But the other version of me is the failed student, sitting at her books, fat and spotty, bored and boring and distinctly unattractive. If I could keep the first "Me" all the time and just let her do a bit of studying when she needed to, I'd get on a lot better, wouldn't I?'

I thought about that for a minute. 'So you're objecting to the idea that you can just learn a bunch of new techniques and that will change the way you've been behaving in certain situations for the last ten years or so?'

Jane looked thoughtful. 'Yes, but there's more to it. What I'm saying is you have to believe that you are a person who can behave differently. It's something to do with your identity. So it goes a bit deeper than just following some new rules. See, what I did in the end was I went back to the slim, fit, successful "Me" and made her study and do your exercises. She could handle that. Everybody's got a successful bit of them somewhere that they can build on, I'm sure of it.'

Friday night came around and Lisa arrived early. 'Let me help you with the chairs. And, by the way, thanks for running me home last week. I must have been crazy to do that class. I stayed in bed all weekend – imagine, me, taking two whole days off! Aren't you impressed?'

I was checking through the handouts. 'I am. Very. How are you feeling now?'

'Fine. I've been doing some gentle exercise the last couple of days, but I think I'll give the aerobics a miss tonight. By the way, have you seen Lewis?'

'No. Haven't you?'

'I thought he'd contact me when I didn't make it to the pub last Friday, but I haven't heard a word.' She wrinkled her nose. 'Oh well, I seem to have a five day maximum limit on relationships at the moment, don't I?'

'What about Mo?' I asked. 'She's the one I'm really worried about. I've got a feeling that you've got life and the universe under control at the moment. Is she coming tonight?'

A lapse does not a relapse make

'I doubt it. I hardly ever see her. She works incredible hours. I think it stops her thinking about things. And she's just eating at her desk I suppose. She certainly never has dinner with me any more. Just when I was starting to make more of an effort. It's, like, she's lost confidence in herself.'

Then it seemed like everybody else arrived at once. Lewis came in at the end on his own. He looked forbidding and he didn't even glance towards Lisa and me, though he had to brush past us to find a seat.

Lisa raised her eyebrows at his back and shrugged. 'See what I mean?' she said and settled herself towards the back of the room.

I was just about to start when Jane walked in. Before she sat down, I called her up to the front. 'I want to introduce you to Jane.' I told them. 'Some of you will recognise her because she works here. I just want her to tell you something.'

'Hey, wait a minute, I'm here to learn with the rest of you.' She protested.

'Get her off,' yelled Faye from the back, 'and if you're letting her stay, at least make her stuff this up her tracksuit so the rest of us don't feel quite so bad.'

To my surprise, Jane walked across, took the rolled up sweater from Faye and did as she was told. She then came back and stood at the front beside me. 'I think I know what Pete's going to ask me. You want me to say why I'm here, right?'

I nodded.

'Well, a couple of months ago, when I was studying for exams and going through a really stressful patch in my life, I gained about ten pounds. It has never happened to me before and I know what went wrong. I stopped exercising and I sat around eating double choc chip cookies.'

'Well,' said Eve, 'you don't look ten pounds overweight to me, or at least you didn't without the padding. Are you going to tell us how you lost it?'

'I think I lost it because I didn't believe I was a fat sort of person. It was a temporary blip for me. Or do I mean blimp? Anyway, I believe I'm really a slim, fit person who likes a lot of exercise, so, once the pressure was off and the exams were over, it was lovely to be able to get back to my old lifestyle – cut out the fat and sugar and get moving again. And my weight went back to normal pretty quickly. It suddenly occurred to me that, if I hadn't had a pretty positive image of myself, it would have been a lot harder to lose that weight. I want to see if I can find out how to make that work for other people. Is that all, Pete?'

'Yes, Jane, thank you.' I turned to the group. 'I wanted to show you an example of how a positive belief can work for you.'

Hey! This is your life, your body, your wellbeing

Next time a bar of chocolate tells you to eat it, tell it to shut up

Jane went to sit down, then she turned back and faced the group again. 'Wait a minute, though. I have negative beliefs too. I believed that I was no good at studying for exams and that the only way to do it was to sit down all day and eat biscuits while I dozed over a pile of books. I can remember a maths teacher telling me I'd better stick to PhysEd because I had more muscle than brainpower. I've never forgotten that.'

'So you're telling us we can cherry pick what we believe about ourselves?' asked Lewis. 'I believe I'm a thirty-something ex rugby player with a weight problem. Now why don't you knock the legs off that one for me.'

'Attitude problem more like,' said Eve, who was sitting next to him. 'And I thought you'd improved lately.'

Lewis turned in his seat and looked at Eve, frowning. He towered over her, even sitting down. 'Go on then. Tell me why I'm not a thirty something male with a weight problem?'

'Don't be daft, Lewis. You know you can't do anything about your age or your gender.'

'Oh, I don't know about that.' Faye looked over her shoulder at Chris who made a face at her and laughed. 'But,' she continued, 'you can do something about the weight problem. Just because you're over thirty, just because you don't kick a ball around any more, just because you're a man, doesn't mean that you have to look like Cyril Smith.'

Lewis happened to be wearing a baggy suit which made him look bigger than he actually was. 'Well, if we're going to be personal about this, just because you're a middle aged woman who can't walk past a cake shop doesn't mean you have to go to parties wearing pink jeans. I don't believe shops should be allowed to sell them in size 20.'

'I am not a size 20. And you are more than half a stone overweight, cheeky sod.'

Jane leaned over to Lisa. 'Is it always like this?'

'Some nights are worse than others. We usually make friends and end up going to the pub afterwards though.'

I clapped my hands for silence. 'Lewis is right. There are some things you can't change. Fortunately your weight is not one of them. You may find it a little more difficult to control as you get older, but that's largely a matter of your lifestyle and expectations. You can change the way you live, the way you eat and what you expect of yourselves.'

'The first step is to flush out your negative beliefs. Every negative belief you carry around is like having a ball and chain around your ankle. These beliefs are just rules and general statements we've made in our lives, that's all they are, not universal truths. Yet they are strong enough to determine how we live and whether we're happy and healthy or sad and stressed. Fortunately, as soon as we challenge the information that supports these negative beliefs, we make them vulnerable to change.

I have not failed 10,000 times, I have successfully found 10,000 ways that will not work.

Thomas Edison

We've installed a doubt. The more we challenge and change the support structure of our beliefs, the more likely it is that the belief itself will wither away. If it's not supported, it will collapse. And once you've collapsed some of your old, negative beliefs, you can make room for some new, positive empowering ones.'

'Hallellujah,' shouted Lewis.

Suddenly, Lisa stood up. 'I've had enough of this. Will you stop interrupting? It's the last group in case you didn't know. Unless you want to sit through the whole bloody eight weeks again, I suggest you pay attention. You do have a problem with your attention span, don't you Lewis?'

Lewis got up and turned around to face her. He leaned menacingly on the back of his chair. 'I have a problem with my attention span? Excuse me but didn't we have an arrangement to meet for a drink last Friday? I sat in the window at the Duke's Head until I noticed you leave the club with Pete. I assumed you were having a bit of private tutoring so I didn't bother to stop you.'

Eve and Faye folded their arms in unison and settled down to enjoy this free display of emotion.

'Blimey,' said Jane, 'it's getting better all the time.'

Lisa blushed and then went pale again. 'Oh. I thought you just meant to go for a drink with everybody else after the group, I didn't know you were waiting for me specially.'

'Well, I was. And I called you Saturday and left God knows how many messages on your answering machine. And Sunday. You didn't even have the courtesy to call me back.'

'I was in bed all day.'

'What?'

'With flu. I was ill, all weekend in fact. I never even hear the phone ring in my room and it's Mo's answering machine anyway.'

Eve nodded vigorously. 'It's true, is that. She looked terrible last week, didn't you, Love? You shouldn't have been out at all. Men never notice things like that.'

'Lisa always looks good to me,' said Lewis. He sat down heavily and put his head in his hands. Faye patted his shoulder. He didn't even snarl at her.

'Well,' I said, 'just to round up on beliefs. I want you all to spend some time thinking about any ideas you may be carrying around that are undermining your weight control programme. When you challenge what's supporting them you often find they weren't even your own ideas in the first place. It may be something your teacher said, or your parents or friends, or enemies, it doesn't matter. If it doesn't empower you, you don't have to live by it.'

SUGAR

Sugar, after fat, is the biggest disrupter of healthy eating, being both high in calories and linked to diabetes, obesity, heart disease, migraines, low immunity, skin disorders, yeast overgrowth and, of course, tooth decay.

Eating Sugar

Buy reduced or sugar-free versions of food and drinks.

When baking, try and half the sugar or use fruit or fresh juice to sweeten.

Check food labels. Sugar often sneaks into food and it's all empty added calories.

White grapes and dried fruits stave off sugar cravings – but they are high calorie.

Buy foods sweetened with juices or fruit.

Health shops have loads of healthy sweet treats - and some unhealthy ones too.

When you have a sweet craving, have something savoury instead. Often it is just our mind playing tricks on us and the body doesn't want sugar at all.

Chris stood up. He didn't need to come to the front in order to get everybody's attention. 'Before we finish, I want to ask Pete about failure. There are some of us here tonight who have already lost most of the weight we set out to lose and there are some of us who are well on the way to success. But what about the ones who aren't going to make it first time around? I'm sure all of us at some time or other are going to have a lapse, or a relapse. Doesn't failure just reinforce our negative beliefs and set us back to where we started?'

'It's not the behaviour, it's the response that matters. So you overeat once in a while. Maybe you go through a period in your life, like Jane did, where you were gaining weight and you felt out of control. That doesn't make you a fat person for the rest of your life. Just learn from it. If what you're doing doesn't work, do something different. In fact,' I told them, 'failures are a useful form of feedback. Think about Kentucky Fried Chicken …'

'I do,' Ben said. 'Far too often.'

'Well, Colonel Sanders was refused 1,009 times before he heard his first YES. Slimming's no different. You may not get your personal eating schedule right first time, you may forget about your Food Cake in times of stress but, if you gain weight, what you do is, you tell yourself, "Try something different". If eating lard and watching TV doesn't seem to be working for you, try something different. Come up with your own formula, your own exercise plan, your own Food Cake. Personalise it.'

'That sounds like hard work,' said Faye. 'Sometimes, you know, I still miss the Miriam approach. The lists she used to give us of things we could do and couldn't do, and we'd just tick them off and get weighed.'

I wondered then, as I've wondered before, why I never manage to bring out all the objections until the very end. I raised my voice to answer, more than I meant to, 'BUT DID YOU LOSE WEIGHT?'

Faye jumped back in her seat. 'No.'

'Alright then. What I'm telling you to do is hard work at first, because it means getting to know yourself and that's difficult enough. But when you do get to know yourself better, when you do become aware of when you're hungry and when you're thirsty and when you learn how to relax and enjoy life more, it will get easier. Even better, you will see results. You already have seen results.'

Before we finished for the evening, I'd already decided not to join them all in the Duke's Head. I planned to go and find Mo and see if I could do anything to help her back on track. 'I may not be able to make it for a drink tonight,' I told them. 'I'll send Jane over instead of me. But I suggest we have a reunion in three weeks. How about it?'

During the re-grouping that followed I saw Faye prod Jane's padded belly. 'You can take that out now.'

'Are you sure? I was trying to think fat.'

SWEET

When you eat a bar of chocolate or a triple layer fudge cake, there is a momentary explosion of pleasure on your taste buds, but your body is left to pick up the pieces.

After the momentary pleasure, you might feel unsatisfied. Yet the fat cells are immediately filled and your blood vessels are eventually left coated and clogged.

A sugar hit puts a great strain on your regulatory system because sugar is absorbed so fast into the bloodstream.

'Well, we're all trying to think thin. Come on, I'll buy you a mineral water. You can have a slice of lemon in it if you like.'

'I'd rather have a pint, without the lemon. I'm not even into designer beer.'

They went out laughing.

I wasn't looking forward to knocking on Mo's door. When I thought back to when it all started at the beginning of the year, how bouncy and carefree she'd been then. I wished she could go back to being the Mo I remembered, even if it meant taking the weight with her. When she opened the door, I could see that she hadn't regained all the weight she'd lost but she seemed to be sagging with unhappiness.

'Aren't you going to ask me in?'

'I suppose so. Why aren't you having a farewell drink with all your successful losers?'

'Success or failure is irrelevant in the short term, Mo. It's your attitude that counts. Didn't anyone ever tell you that successful people relish mistakes because they give them the opportunity to learn and to do something different next time? You and I both know that there are going to be times when you are faced with difficult circumstances, so the question is not whether you are going to have knock backs, but rather how you deal with them.'

'I can apply that to business but I'm not sure it works in terms of emotional turmoil and losing weight.'

'Why didn't you come tonight?'

'I've got too much on my mind to worry about a weight control group at the moment.' She paused. 'Was Chris there?'

'Yes.'

'Did he say anything?'

'Not really. Has he been in touch?'

'He may have left messages on the answering machine. I haven't listened to it for a week. I use my mobile for business so I don't have to worry about missing important calls.'

'Do you fancy coming out for a pizza?'

'Is that helpful? When I'm trying to lose weight?'

'You're not trying to lose weight. You gave up, you just said so. Have you already eaten?'

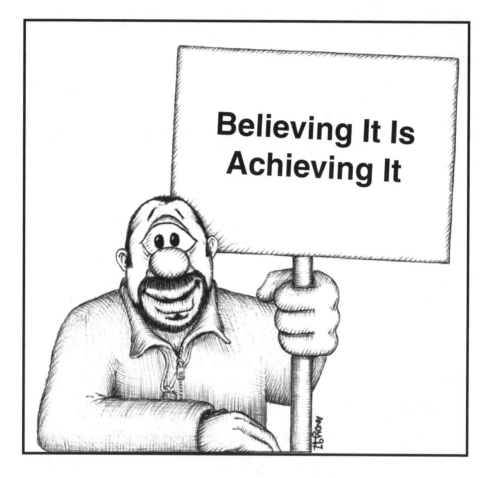

'No, I haven't and I haven't been grazing either. The last couple of days I've been back on the food cake and I've started contributing to the Fat Jar. In fact, there might be enough in it by now to buy us a pizza. I'll come out with you on one condition.'

'What's that.'

'That you don't try and cheer me up.'

We'd only been in the restaurant ten minutes when I felt a draught and looked up. My heart sank. The Lighten Up group were trooping in, making a lot of noise. I looked again and counted. Chris wasn't with them. Neither was Ben. Neither were Lisa and Lewis. I glanced across at Mo who had stiffened and was checking them out like me. Faye and Eve broke away from the rest and came over to our table.

Faye put her arms round Mo. 'We've been so worried about you, Sweetheart.'

'Running away never solved anything,' added Eve. Unhelpfully.

Mo smiled. 'I figured that out. And, what's more, I did it before I'd even had time to regain all the weight I'd lost. How about you two? Have you reached your target weight?'

'I don't know,' Eve admitted. 'I took Pete seriously and gave the scales to my sister-in-law. They were these new digital ones and she fell for it. I'm hoping she'll have gained at least a stone before my daughter's wedding. She always upstages me at family dos.'

'How about a glass of wine?' Faye suggested. She looked at me nervously.

'I'm not going to stop you drinking wine. I'll have a glass myself. Just make sure you taste it, drink it slowly and enjoy it. We're celebrating tonight, not drowning our sorrows. Right?'

The next week I started a new Lighten Up class. They were nothing like as lively as the previous group. 'That last lot were a real bunch of characters, weren't they?' said Jane, one lunchtime. 'Are the Lighten Up classes always that hectic?'

'No. Thank goodness.' She looked surprised.

'It's all very well if you're in the audience,' I told her, 'but it's very tiring when they challenge every single thing you tell them.' I knew I'd learned a lot from them though. And, as it happened, I still had a lot more to learn.

Before I knew it, the night of the Lighten Up reunion at the Duke's Head came around. I thought we had a full turn-out but my heart sank when I looked around and realised Mo was missing again.

'Where's Mo?' I whispered to Lisa.

DO YOU BELIEVE YOU CAN BE SLIMMER?

Some beliefs have firmer foundations than others.

If you believe you can be slimmer, what is supporting that? What are you doing that's moving you in the right direction?

Are you:

> writing down what you eat?
> exercising?
> being positive?
> eating a balanced diet?
> thinking before you shop?
> cutting down on FAT?
> slowing down your eating?
> choosing more nutritious foods?
> drinking plenty of water?
> thinking before you eat?
> eating when you're hungry?
> including plenty of fruit and vegetables?

'She couldn't face Chris and she's had a bad week. You know, lots of business lunches, lots of snacky evenings and lots of depression. It seems to have hit her again. And I'm afraid she's gained weight. I can see it.'

I stood up to welcome everybody back and offered to buy them a drink. 'No, we'll get the first round – we've all been raiding our Fat Jars,' said Faye.

When everybody had settled down I told them my idea. 'What about a Midsummer outing?'

'What, like a long weekend in Benidorm?' suggested Faye.

'Well, you're right about the seaside.' I opened my rucksack and pulled out a poster for the London to Brighton Bike Ride on June 21st. 'How about it?'

There was a moment's silence. Then Chris started laughing.

Eve was the first to find her voice. 'You're barmy, you are, that must be fifty miles at least.'

'Fifty six from Clapham Common,' I told her, 'but we don't have to rush. We can start early and take our time. Picnic on the beach when we get there. We can arrange a point to meet in case anybody gets lost.'

'In case anybody gets left behind, you mean,' said Faye.

Lisa was enthusiastic. 'It's a great idea, I've been thinking I'm ready for a longer run.'

Lewis protested. 'I haven't got a bike.' He looked at Lisa. 'Why don't we get a tandem?'

'Don't be silly, Lewis. Serious style error. Plus I will end up doing all the pedalling for both of us. You are congenitally lazy.'

Everybody was still so fascinated by the explosive potential of the Lisa and Lewis partnership that we all waited for the response. Lewis just smiled at Lisa and took a sip of his beer. Everybody else breathed out.

'Disappointing,' muttered Chris.

'It's my round,' said Ben. 'Are you drinking halves, Lewis?'

Lewis shrugged. 'Looks like it, doesn't it? You can laugh but since this lady took control of my life I've lost five pounds and I'm back to running four days a week.'

Chris frowned at him. 'You look to me like you lost a lot more than five pounds. I suppose Madam doesn't let you get on the scales?'

'There are scales at the gym. It's more than just weight loss, I'm getting some of the muscle back.'

Mistakes are not failures. They are lessons for success.

Lisa patted his shoulder. 'It's very impressive,' she said sweetly.

'In fact,' Lewis added, 'we found a couple of suits I hadn't been able to wear for at least four years and they fit me again, don't they Lisa?'

'Did fit you. I gave them to the charity shop. Just because you can wear out-of-date clothes doesn't mean I'll actually let you do it.'

'Well,' said Chris, 'now that we're getting down to life's essentials, let's do some real strategic planning for this outing. The point is, 'What are we going to wear?' Obviously we need team T-shirts, but I refuse to cycle to Brighton in something that says "Diet Group" on it.'

'Or anything pink,' added Faye.

'Or anything that doesn't match Chris's bike, I suspect,' said Lisa, cattily.

Ben appeared with a tray of drinks. 'You'll never guess who's just walked in. Up at the bar there. It's Miriam and the group from St Mark's.'

I looked over and waved at Miriam. She waved back and a couple of minutes later the entire St Mark's slimming group had joined us. 'Where have you all been?' she asked. 'I haven't seen any of you for the last couple of Friday nights.'

'Oh, the new group doesn't go to the Duke's Head,' I told her.

'New group?'

'This is just a reunion. My Lighten Up classes run for eight weeks, then they're on their own.'

'But what if they don't lose all the weight they want to lose in eight weeks?'

'I didn't lose much,' Faye told her. 'I've lost a lot more steadily since the meetings finished. We'd got all the information we needed, and it was just a question of applying it to our own bodies, if you see what I mean.'

'Sounds like nicotine patches. Something you just stick on,' Miriam said, sceptically.

'No,' Eve shook her head. 'How it works is that the ideas sort of sink in and become like part of you. A lot of the little mental exercises we've practised get to be kind of automatic. It all kind of seeps in gradually and by then, you've already changed and there's no going back.'

'Some people might call that brainwashing.'

'Miriam, you're a professional pessimist,' I said.

'Of course I am. That's why I get repeat business and you don't.'

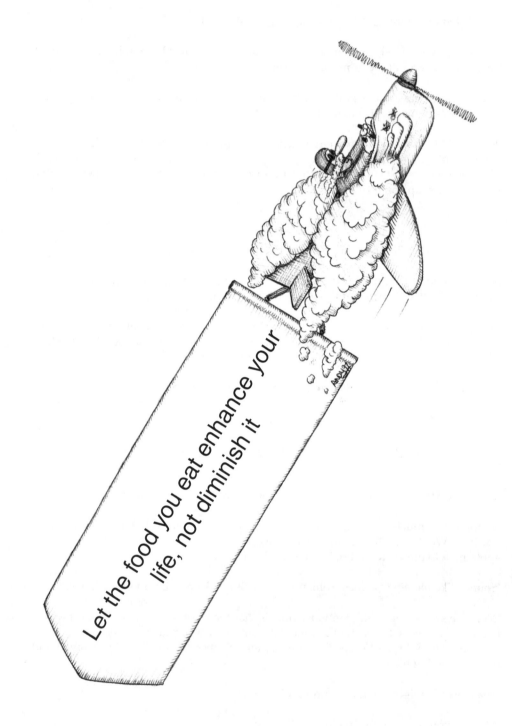

Let the food you eat enhance your life, not diminish it

'You're making a profit out of loss, Miriam. And it's not weight loss. It's loss of self esteem. What Pete teaches isn't brainwashing. It's the opposite. It's about starting to believe you can be how you want to be without relying on somebody else to tell you what you can do and what you can't,' said Lisa.

Lewis looked adoringly at her. 'Well I haven't made it yet in that case, because I'm relying on you to have enough self belief for both of us.'

Everybody groaned and there were some catcalls from the back.

Lisa looked embarrassed and pushed him away. Miriam spotted a weak moment and homed in like a cruise missile. 'Oh, Lisa, I didn't see you there. Tell me, Dear, how's your friend Mo? I heard some rumours that she wasn't well.'

But Miriam had met her match. 'She's fine,' Lisa told her casually, 'just working too hard at the moment. It's the wedding season and that means her business is flat out at weekends as well as during the week. She did a family wedding for you last year, didn't she, Miriam? How is your daughter these days? I hope she's managing to stick to the diet now that she's not so closely supervised.'

I will say this for Miriam. She'll never back down from a challenge. 'My family are all fine, thank you, ' she said, 'And I'm glad to hear that Mo is well too. It's funny though because I heard she'd put on a bit of weight lately.' She stood up and looked around, very pointedly. 'I can't seem to see her here tonight.'

As soon as she stood up, Chris spotted her. He put down his wineglass and came across. He's quite impressive, even when he isn't wearing high heels and Miriam shrank back a little.

He put his hand on her shoulder. 'Miriam. How lovely to see you. We haven't had a chance to talk since we did our double act here, have we? I was wondering if you had a theatrical background, and then, when I saw you a few weeks ago with that cake, I just thought to myself, "with timing like that, she's just got to be in the business".'

We could all see that he had her on the ropes. She was looking past him for a clear way out, but the pub was packed. 'I was on the stage for a while,' she said. 'We must talk sometime, but I have to rush now.'

One of the ladies from the St Mark's group came up. 'What happened to Miriam? She buys us all a diet coke and then does a runner, leaving us exposed to temptation.'

'If there's any temptation going around here I'm giving in to it first,' said Faye, who obviously knew quite a few of Miriam's losers.

'And if you mean Chris and Ben,' added Eve, 'you're out of luck. Stick to the peanuts, that's my advice. Satisfaction guaranteed.'

Another one of the St Mark's contingent laughed, 'We're not allowed peanuts anyway so it looks like it's another diet coke or an evening back at home plotting tomorrow's calorie allowance.'

Don't take your eyes off the goal

**Hyrum Smith,
Inventor of the Day Planner**

'Well, here's something even Miriam can't object to. Why don't you all join forces with us and do the London to Brighton Bike Ride?'

There was some raucous laughter, followed pretty quickly by some serious interest among the younger ones. Chris seemed to have taken the project to heart so I left him to get on with organising the important stuff like T-shirts and picnics. I leaned over and shouted in his ear, 'Tell me when you need some input from me.' He nodded.

Before I left, I sat down with Lisa and Lewis for a few minutes. 'I'm just going,' I told them. 'Do you think it would be alright for me to call on Mo or does she want to be alone?'

'Give her another week. She doesn't seem to want to talk to anybody at the moment.' Lisa said. 'I'll tell you something else that's worrying me. She's taken to drinking on her own in the evening. And I know she's drinking wine at lunchtime too. She never used to do that.'

'While you solve Mo's problems, why don't I get another round in,' Lewis suggested.

Lisa put her arm round his neck. 'You don't really want another drink, do you Lewis? Now think carefully, what do you want?'

Faye leaned across. 'No wonder he's losing weight if he's being deprived of five pints a night. What he needs now is a really interesting displacement activity to stop him thinking about the beer.'

Everybody heard that one and the noise level rose again.

I stood up to go. 'Even if you're only keeping him away from one pint a night,' I told Lisa, 'it's still a lot of calories. And if Mo's drinking that probably explains some of her weight gain as well.'

'I've got an idea,' shouted Eve. 'Why don't we observe the five minute rule between drinks?'

'Sorry to disappoint you, but it's a fifty minute rule with wine and beer.'

I got out nearly as fast as Miriam. On the way home, I wondered whether the London to Brighton idea was such a good one. Too late to think that now, they were already off and pedalling. So to speak.

Chapter 12

The Difference That Makes The Difference

One evening after the Lighten Up reunion, Chris arrived at the club. He waved a bunch of forms at me. 'These are for the London to Brighton, Pete. Can you give me the Lighten Up address list so I can send them out? We need to get everybody together for a practice run.'

'You mean we're going to do it twice?'

'No, we're just going to ride round the park for the next three weekends. Everybody who can manage that should be able to get to Brighton. It's just so that people know what it feels like to do more than a couple of miles. Like a rehearsal. What do you think about Sunday afternoons?'

'That sounds good. I'll put a notice up on the board here as well. By the way, what did you decide about T-shirts?'

'Well, I thought we'd have shocking pink and 'Pete Cohen – Keep Going' picked out in gold sequins.'

'It's lucky for you that you're bigger than me,' I told him. 'Otherwise I might feel obliged to smack you in the teeth. As it is, Faye will probably do it for me if you go ahead with that idea.'

'Don't worry. We'll settle for plain white with "Lighten Up and Get a Life" on the back and we thought we'd all try to get sponsors so we can raise money as a team for the British Heart Research Foundation.'

I couldn't argue with that. Later on, I was queuing up at the local Seven Eleven when Miriam came up and stood behind me. She had a bottle of skimmed milk and some low fat spread in her hand. 'Hello, Peter. How's your London to Brighton team shaping up?'

I had to look twice. She was actually wearing shorts and a T-shirt. She still had the earrings and the hairdo though. 'What do you mean?'

'Well, my group are doing it too, you know. They told me last week that you'd invited us to join you which is very kind, but I feel that an outing like this really needs proper organisation.' She paused, 'I don't believed you've started your training programme yet, have you Peter? I've been taking my team round the park twice a week for the last fortnight. Oh, and I hope you're raising plenty of money for the Heart Foundation, because some of your people look as if they're going to need the cardiac emergency unit. Especially if they carry on patronising the Duke's Head instead of getting out on two wheels.'

LAPSING, RELAPSING AND COLLAPSING

One of **my** most important messages is for each of you to be able to distinguish between a **Lapse,** a **Relapse** and a total **Collapse**.

Lapses and Relapses are nothing to worry about. They are just behaviour patterns.

A Lapse is a slight error or slip, a discreet event, like eating crisps and peanuts *all night* at a party, or a whole tub of ice cream one lonely evening at home, or getting up too late to walk to work for a few days. It doesn't matter. Once it's done (or not done) it's over with.

A Relapse is when you manage to string a whole series of lapses together so that it starts to look like the state you were in before you started changing.

A Collapse happens when you fall back into your old behaviour patterns and start believing again your old negative beliefs about yourself, when you feel like it's not worth bothering to change any more or when you find you get just as much satisfaction from whining about your weight as from being slim.

'Ah, but wait till you see our T-shirts,' I said.

She turned around. Written across her back was 'Miriam's Miracle Diet' and her phone number.

'Well, that's one way to get dates, I suppose.'

She waved a finger at me. 'No respect. That's the trouble with young people today! Let's see how we do on June 21st.'

'It's not a race. In fact, why don't we all agree to meet on the sea front and picnic together? That could be fun. You and Chris could round off the day by doing a little cabaret at the end of the pier.'

For a minute my fate was in the balance. Then she laughed. 'We'll see. Anyway, you're holding up the queue. And that Magnum's going to melt unless you start licking soon.'

I walked thoughtfully back down the street. It was obviously time I got involved with the arrangements for the Midsummer outing. It sounded as though Miriam was running her team like a military operation and over the past few months I'd become only too well aware of my Lighten Up group's tendency to go AWOL at a moment's notice. I also knew very well that, while some of them still tended to under-estimate their abilities, some of the others were frighteningly unaware of their own limits. As usual my imagination started to take over and pretty soon I had a clear picture of them setting off dressed like a designer fashion team and getting drunk, bingeing or falling over before they even got to the North Downs. I had quite a bit of respect for Chris's charisma, cooking and fashion sense, but his organisational skills had yet to be proved.

Next thing I knew I was outside Mo and Lisa's flat. I hadn't intended to visit but there I was. So I rang the bell.

Lisa opened the door. 'Come in, we were just talking about you.' I could hear male voices behind her.

When I got into the kitchen Chris and Ben were sitting at the kitchen table sorting out forms and address labels. Chris looked up. 'I decided to get some help with the envelopes. I didn't realise you were coming over – I could have given you a lift.'

'That's funny. I was just walking along thinking I'd better get involved in planning this thing. It's not fair to leave it all to you when it was my idea in the first place.'

Lisa put a hand on both the men's shoulders. They looked up at her and burst out laughing. I felt totally excluded.

'What's the joke?'

'Before you arrived we were just laying bets about how long it would be before you decided to interfere, sorry, help. You don't trust us an inch, do you?'

The chains of habit are too weak to be felt until they are too strong to be broken

Samuel Johnson

'Well, thinking back to a few memorable moments over the past few months, I think I've got good reasons to feel you need a little support.'

'If you mean supervision, say so.'

I remembered the conversation with Miriam. 'Alright then. Not supervision. Leadership. And I know something you don't.'

They looked at me.

'Miriam's group are going to do it as well. They've been practising for weeks and their T-shirts are already printed.'

There was a minute's respectful silence while we all made our own pictures of Miriam and her team cycling triumphantly into Brighton in perfect formation, their T-shirts immaculate and their make-up colour co-ordinated. Then Lisa made a move. She switched on the kettle and reached for the teabags. 'Well, this is getting serious.'

'What are their T-shirts like. Have you seen them?' Chris asked anxiously.

'To hell with their T-shirts. I haven't even got a bicycle yet. And the whole school seems to be sponsoring me.' Ben looked distraught.

'This isn't a race or any kind of competition,' I reminded them. 'It's just for fun. It's about getting out and about in the fresh air and exercising your body.'

Lisa handed round the mugs and sat down. 'Speaking of which, I feel exhausted. I haven't felt this low since I had flu a couple of weeks ago.'

Ben frowned at her 'You look tired – how come you get 'flu in the spring anyway? Everybody else gets it in winter.'

'It was the trauma of breaking up with you I expect.'

Ben looked embarrassed and Chris answered for him. 'You can't break up something that never got started. Anyway, where's Lewis tonight?'

'We go to judo together on Tuesdays. Normally I really enjoy it – it's a great way to channel your aggression. Imagine, me enjoying exercise! But tonight I didn't feel up to it, so I sent Lewis on his own – and I don't feel bad about it. I know tomorrow I'll be back on form again.' She patted Ben's shoulder. 'There you are, see what a lucky escape you had. I could have been nagging you instead of Lewis.'

'At least he'll be fit for the bike ride,' Ben said gloomily.

'So will you. You've been taking more exercise since the beginning of the Lighten Up group. Maybe not as much as if I'd been in charge of you, but you're looking better and better all the time.'

Success is on the other side of failure

**T J Watson,
Founder of IBM**

While she was talking to Ben, I was watching Lisa carefully. I thought back to that session at the club in the New Year. Five months ago. It didn't seem possible. She was tired tonight, but she didn't have that fragile transparency I'd noticed then. She looked a strong healthy young woman and this time it had nothing to do with make-up. 'Last January, you'd have dragged yourself to judo anyway, Lisa. Could it be that you're starting to listen to your body instead of overriding it and pushing yourself too hard like you used to?'

'If I wake up feeling low I don't ignore it any more. I ask myself why. And if I get an answer that makes sense I do something about it. When I know I haven't had enough sleep I don't push myself to do a workout. A few weeks ago I'd have done the workout even if I was ill, let alone just tired.'

Ben suddenly became animated. 'It's a matter of respect. Respect yourself. I can relate to that. I just thought it was more of a psychological thing than a physical one,' he added.

Lisa was thoughtful 'I didn't feel like respecting my body, it was more like living with the enemy. I was so sure it was going to let me down and get fat if I relaxed for a minute that I spent years trying to silence it. And I got very good at silencing it. The trouble is, once you start to listen to your body again, it isn't so easy to switch off. It feels right. It's insidious. As long as I thought, "well, I've got a body but it's not the one I want", I felt free to mistreat it. It's hard to respect yourself physically when you feel like that.'

Ben interrupted, 'Your body is a temple not a dustbin.'

'That's a good one, where did you hear that?' I asked him.

He laughed 'You can have the copyright for a small fee. My Sunday School teacher told me that when I used to eat sweets in church. I hadn't heard it for years but I thought of it again when I started writing down what I was eating and looking for patterns. That's when I noticed I was definitely not being good to myself. I used to eat when I wasn't hungry, I didn't bother to taste my food – I was starving myself when my body was crying out for a sandwich or a bowl of cereal.'

'I remember denying myself an apple,' Lisa said. 'That was a turning point for me when I wrote that down. An apple, for God's sake. I'd eaten all kinds of junk the night before. Major fat and sugar binge and then I wouldn't let myself eat the piece of fruit I really wanted twelve hours later.'

'When you've had a night like that, Lisa, you need to be even nicer to your body than usual. That doesn't mean starving it. It means feeding it with what it wants when it's good and ready. When you've put yourself under nutritional stress, give yourself time to recover.'

'I've learned that, Pete. I know that now. I think that's why "Think Before You Eat" was one of the fastest habits I ever learned. It's what my body wanted me to do anyway, so I didn't really have to learn it. It's so embedded now that it happens in my

STRESS

There are two ways of dealing with stress, Quick Fixes and Relaxation.

Quick Fixes

Smoking. Feels like a relaxant but actually a stimulant. Expensive, smelly and damaging to the health.

Alcohol. A depressant. Expensive, smelly and damaging to the health.

Caffeine. The stimulant in the three most popular drinks (apart from alcohol) worldwide: cola, coffee & tea. It won't relax you but it's not quite as disastrous health-wise as smoking and alcohol.

Over-eating and under-eating. Has no effect on stress other than to add to it by causing weight gain or illness.

O*verwork. Has a short-term distracting effect but increases stress in the long term.

Drugs. Expensive and may be damaging to health and relationships.

None of the these will cure stress. All of them will take your mind off it briefly. In the long term they actually increase the pressure and some of them will also make you ill.

mind whether I want it to or not. I can go out at lunchtime thinking "salad and Ryvita" and I come back with a chicken sandwich and an orange. It's more than respecting your body, it's trusting your instincts. And I don't even get so many mega-cravings any more.'

'So you're almost at the unconscious competence stage?' I asked her.

'The what?'

'Remember the last Lighten Up group? We were talking about how you go through these stages of learning something. Like when you start to drive, and because you've been driven about by somebody else all your life, you think you just get in a car and it goes. Well, that's Unconscious Incompetence.'

Ben covered his face with his hands. 'I remember my first driving lesson. I got in the driver's seat. I switched on the engine and it was in gear so it stalled straight away. Then my brother told me I had to check for neutral, check the mirrors, the handbrake, get the clutch down while I changed gear … I just got out and I said to him, "This is ridiculous. I am never going to be able to do all this at the same time", and he was laughing so much …'

'I think that's the "Conscious Incompetence stage", am I right?' Lisa looked at me. I nodded.

'But, after a couple of lessons,' Ben continued, 'I could get up to third gear and go round the car park but I had to think about every move I made, it was really hard work. It was weeks before I could actually change gear properly and use the signals and everything else without consciously telling myself what to do.'

'That's exactly it,' I told them. 'It's the same with learning any new techniques. While you've got to think "Now I've got to do Think Before You Eat" or "It's time to put something in the Fat Jar", it's all a bit of an effort. But when you get to the stage where your subconscious is doing it all for you - that's when your new, slender self can go out and play.' Even as I said it, I was thinking to myself that this particular Lighten Up group had probably taken themselves out to play faster than any of the others I'd worked with. Except for Mo of course, it was almost as if she'd un-learned all the good things she'd once known.

I suddenly realised that Lisa was still talking to me. Sorry, Lisa, what was that?'

She looked at me suspiciously. 'Your mind was somewhere else, obviously. I was just saying that I'm starting to find it easy to do things that used to be really hard. I even got weighed at the Well Woman clinic last week and that's the first time I've been near any scales in a couple of months. I used to weigh myself all the time at home, but I dreaded going for my check up because it meant somebody else was looking at my weight.'

Chris patted her on the back. 'Congratulations. You've come a long way. How light are you?'

RELAXATION

Relaxation is the only sure-fire, long-term method of coping with stress. It's cheap, it's not anti-social and it doesn't damage your health.

Identify your personal pressure points.

Select the relaxation techniques which work for you.

Practice them until they become an automatic response.

She pulled a face. Actually, I'm about four pounds over the weight I thought I needed to be. But everything fits me and I feel good. I'm not going to lose any sleep over it.'

The door slammed and Lewis walked in. I hadn't seen him for a few weeks. "What a difference," I thought to myself. I'd known Ben when he was in good shape, but I'd never seen Lewis looking like anything but a belligerent slob.

Lewis stopped in the doorway and scowled at us. 'What the hell is going on here? Why are all these people in the kitchen, Lisa?' The change was obviously skin deep. Not much of a personality change in evidence so far.

'Isn't judo supposed to channel your aggression?' I asked him.

Lisa gave me a warning look and put her arm round him. 'It's my kitchen and they're your friends. We're just planning the bike ride. Chris brought the forms round.'

Lewis shrugged, then he leaned across to Ben and tapped him lightly in the middle. 'Just breathing in won't get rid of that. How's the training going? Have you got a bike yet?'

Ben looked at him scornfully. 'I've got plenty of time.'

Chris stuck the last label onto the last envelope. 'We're ready to start stuffing them now.'

'Are you talking about Miriam's diet group again?' I couldn't resist it.

'No, but it's not a bad idea. After all, that's what she tried to do to us at your party.'

'This is not a competition, how many times do I have to tell you! Pushing yourself to race to Brighton under far from ideal conditions when you haven't trained for it is crazy.'

'Stop lecturing us Pete, we're only joking. Why don't you stop talking and give us a hand.'

I'd already realised I was going to have to scrap my plans for an early night so I sat down at the table. 'I'll help you with this, but I think we'd better put a note in with each form asking everybody to turn up for the first practice this Sunday afternoon.'

We'd nearly finished when Mo arrived. 'I thought it was judo tonight, Lisa. What's going on?'

Lisa smiled at her. 'Come and join us. We're sending out the London to Brighton forms and a notice about the first practice next Sunday.'

Mo shook her head and started backing out of the door. 'I'm going to bed early. I'll leave you to it.'

Lewis sniffed. 'Hang on, I can smell curry. Have you got a takeaway there?'

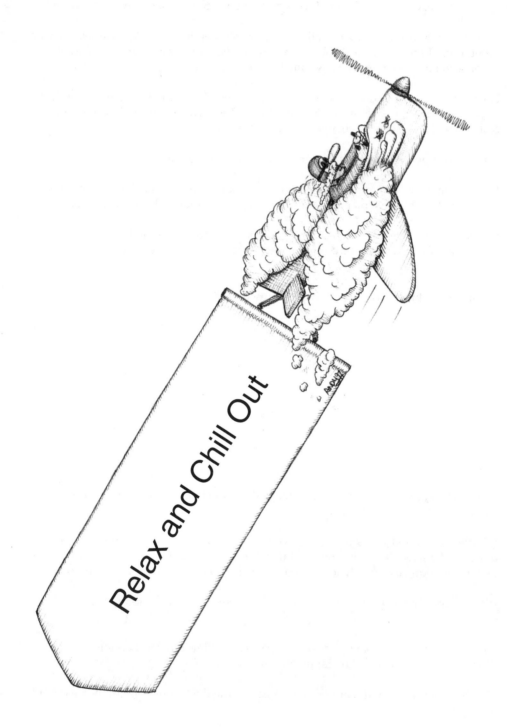

Relax and Chill Out

Mo disappeared and we heard her bedroom door slam.

'You shouldn't have mentioned that,' Lisa told him. 'You just embarrassed her. She always brings takeaways home now but she usually eats in her room because she doesn't like to admit it. I've given up asking if she wants me to cook for her.'

'I suppose you all think this is my fault,' said Chris defensively.

Lisa rounded on him. 'Well you didn't help.'

'Mo had a self-esteem problem anyway. She was just hiding behind the cuddly loveable Mo image. She wanted to be a vamp and I helped her achieve her ambition.'

'Yes and now she's in a worse position than she was before. She can't go back to being plump and happy again. You showed her another way to be and now she's caught in no man's land.'

'No woman's land,' said Chris.

This time Lisa turned round in her chair and faced him. 'Well, isn't that typical! You won't be serious about anything. Not even other people's feelings. Just because life's one big stage performance for you doesn't mean you have a right to assume it's just as surreal for everybody else. Other people have feelings you know.'

Chris looked stunned but before he could defend himself Ben stepped in for him. 'It's time you took more responsibility yourself, Lisa. You were the one who started Mo on the slippery slope to calorie counting. You were her role model. She always wanted to be glamorous like you and you showed her how you did it. Unfortunately she only learned how to make herself miserable. She didn't really get the hang of being thin.'

'When you've all quite finished blaming each other for the state Mo's in, doesn't it occur to you that it might be more constructive to see what you can do to help her?'

We all looked at Lewis in surprise. He continued. 'One thing I've learned from Pete is that you have to take responsibility for yourself and your own body. Nobody else is going to. All you ever get from other people is rules and distractions. Your mum wants you to have second helpings of pudding, Miriam wants you to promise her personally that you'll never touch another treacle tart in your life. Your friends want you to go out and get lagered up like you always did, your girlfriend wants you to eat lettuce…' Lisa looked indignant but he continued. 'None of it's helping you, is it? I don't like to admit it, but taking the time to work out whether you're hungry or not, makes a lot more sense. But you have to do it for yourself.'

He was speaking with passion now. He paused and then thumped his fist on the table. 'People think I'm aggressive, but I only say what I think. Most people are afraid to speak their minds, either to themselves or anyone else.' He turned to Chris. 'Maybe Mo really did think you were the answer to a maiden's prayer. But if she did, then I must say, she really has only herself to blame for what happened.'

Chris frowned. 'I don't like the sound of that, but I can't be bothered to work it out.'

You are what you repeatedly do

Aristotle

'And what was that about lettuce?' Lisa was looking very hard at Lewis. 'I never tried to make you eat lettuce.'

'I don't know about you and Lewis,' Ben said suddenly, 'but I remember that night I took you out to dinner, you went on and on about some fibre diet and that was even after you'd thrown all your slimming books away. I had to wait while you read the whole menu and tried to work out the ingredients.'

'Well, if you'd been more interesting I wouldn't have had to amuse myself with the menu, would I? Anyway, I was just winding you up. Men hate it when you talk about fibre during dinner. You took everything I said so seriously I got bored with myself.'

Chris was laughing at her. 'With attitudes like that you can hardly expect to call me superficial and get away with it.'

I could see that Ben was looking upset, so I decided to lighten the tone a little. 'Fibre's important,' I said, 'but it can be embarrassing if you suddenly up your fibre intake. Your body will react loudly. It has to be a gradual thing.'

'Oh, be quiet for a minute, Pete,' said Ben. 'Fibre's got nothing to do with it.'

'There's gratitude for you,' I thought.

'I didn't mean to be rude,' he went on, 'I'm not as direct as Lewis, but this is really something I always knew. When I let myself get really out of shape, I hated it because I felt I wasn't being fair to myself. You are right about your body letting you know what's right. You've got to listen to yourself, give yourself some time. Your body is a mirror of your inner thoughts and actions. If you love yourself and take care of yourself you will reap the reward.'

Lisa looked at him with frank admiration. 'That's the sensitive side of you that attracted me. I haven't met many men who understand that sort of thing.'

Lewis shook his head in despair. 'Bullshit, Lisa. It was the chocolate cake, remember? Sometimes they look better than they taste. You know what you're always saying to me? Stick to the complex carbohydrates.'

When I walked home, an hour or so later, I was still more worried about the emotional stability of my group than I was about their physical ability to make it from London to Brighton.

On Sunday, of course, it was raining. It wasn't cold but it certainly was wet. I got to the meeting point in the park early but Lisa and Lewis weren't far behind. Lewis was on a mountain bike that wasn't new but looked as though it had cost a fortune.

We had quite a good turnout but Mo was missing. I had a word with Lewis and Lisa who were going on to visit friends after the practice. So I knew Mo would be on her own. When everybody had gone I went round to her flat and rang the bell and hammered on the door. Then I yelled through the letterbox. 'Open this door, Mo. I know you're in there.' I didn't, but it did the trick.

All you are doing is rediscovering your natural relationship with food

She stood on the doorstep. She was wearing the bin-liner tracksuit she'd worn at the first aerobic session. Her face looked sad and puffy. 'What do you want?'

'That usually means 'Oh, alright, come in, seeing as you're here.'

'Come in if you like,' she muttered and turned away. 'I don't care.'

'How much further down are you planning to go?' I asked her.

'Planning? Don't be a cosmic schmuck, Pete, nobody plans to feel this bad.'

'Feeling that bad takes some effort. You have to make sure you're asking yourself stupid questions, for a start. How often do you say to yourself "why do I always fall for the wrong person?", "why am I letting myself go like this?", "why don't things work out for me?".'

She looked me in the eye. 'Because from where I am, they seem like perfectly reasonable questions, that's why.'

'Well if you go on asking yourself depressing questions like that your mind is going to waste a lot of useful brain time looking for answers. It doesn't want to let you down so it rummages around among all your bad memories and comes up with lots of "for instances". Am I right?'

She nodded.

'Well, if you insist on sitting at home talking yourself in circles instead of getting on your bike and joining us in the park, why not ask yourself some useful questions?'

'Like what?'

'Like "What can I do today to get myself back into shape again?" or "How can I make myself look better and feel better?" Or "What have I got in my life that makes me go on making an effort?" – and don't tell me there isn't anything because if that was true you wouldn't even get up in the morning.'

Mo fished in her pocket for a tissue and blew her nose. 'Look, Pete, I understand what you're trying to do and I appreciate it. I've even heard what you're saying. But I need some time to get back on my feet. I've got to do it myself this time.'

I turned to go. Then something occurred to me. 'That's exactly it, isn't it? That's what I'm asking you to do. I'm not offering you a solution or a set of rules.'

She stood in the doorway looking at me. 'Come back in for a minute.' She turned around and I followed her in. The kitchen was littered with books, papers, two large empty kettle chip bags and half a packet of matzos. I picked the cat off one of the chairs so I could sit on it and noticed that it had been asleep on a partly-eaten Snickers bar. 'The cat's covered in chocolate.'

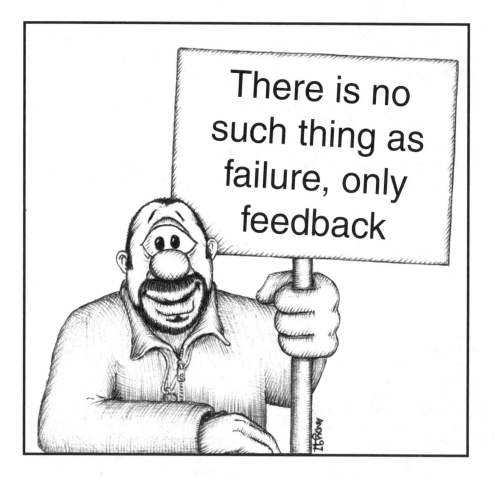

'It's alright. He likes it. He'll wash when he realises.'

Mo took him from me and stuffed him through the cat flap. It was still raining and he looked pretty indignant. She came back and sat down. 'You know, the worst of it is, I was kind of getting the hang of a new way of life. I'd really started to believe I could be slim and attractive and happy.'

'And now you've given up on all three? How about getting them back one at a time? But add a new one, just for practice, until you get the hang of it. How about "I'm a successful business woman", for starters?'

Mo wrinkled her nose. 'You mean "I'm a workaholic", don't you?'

'See, you've made it negative again. Turn it around. I'll give you some suggestions, but they won't work unless you believe them.' I walked over to the whiteboard on the kitchen wall. 'Do you want this shopping list? I'm sure it's the same one that was there last time I came.'

'It's an old list.'

'Right, Mo, let's start with a new one.' I picked up a board marker and wrote:

"I am a successful businesswoman"
"I am attractive"
"I am getting slimmer"
"I am feeling more positive about myself every day"

'Now, come on Mo, look at these. You are not allowed to rub them out unless you replace them with some even more positive ones, or until you have repeated them to yourself every day for a fortnight.'

She was laughing. Just a little bit. But she still threw me out.

I wasn't sure as I walked away from the flat whether I was glad I'd called or not.

On the morning of the bike ride the weather was beautiful. It was a clear, bright, morning and the weather forecast was for a hot day later on. We'd all agreed to meet half a mile from the start at six am. I didn't have much confidence about everybody making it much before half seven but we'd agreed that anyone who didn't turn up by then would make their own way and meet us at the West Pier during the afternoon. Several of us had mobile phones with us so we could stay in touch.

Lisa and Lewis were first to arrive. 'Where's Mo?' I asked.

'She didn't come in last night. She said something about visiting her mum and dad,' Lisa told me. 'I'm really worried about her.'

'No kidding,' I said.

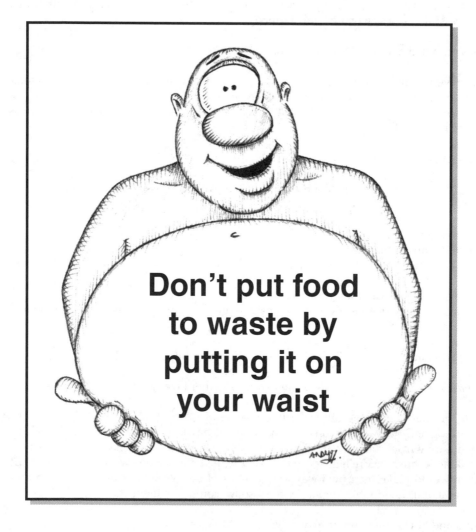

Just then I noticed Faye was on her own. 'Where's Eve?'

'She chickened out at the last minute. She's been doing the park runs but she didn't think she could manage 56 miles all in one go. If you ask me, she was just afraid of holding everybody up. And those two daughters of hers have been teasing her about it.'

'Will you be alright, Faye?'

'Of course I will, Sweetheart. I've done my affirmations and my outcomes and I'm ready for anything. Just save me some champagne if you get there before me?'

'Champagne?' I thought. But it was just a passing thought. Mainly I felt sad. No Eve. And of course, no Mo.

Jane arrived with a contingent from the club and by seven thirty we had everybody except Chris and Ben. 'We'll have to go without them. They know the mobile numbers and the meeting points. Are you all ready to go for the start line?'

'Wait a minute, Pete, I think I can see Ben,' Faye shaded her eyes, 'And Chris. Yes, it couldn't be anyone else.'

My heart sank. With good reason. Chris and Ben appeared, walking their bikes across the traffic lights at the corner.

Chris was wearing an outfit I'd seen before. On stage. Mini-skirt, fishnet tights and high heels and a very convincing wig. Fortunately he was riding a ladies bike. Ben was keeping a five yard distance between them, ignoring Chris's orders to keep up. He looked mortally embarrassed. 'Don't blame me, it wasn't my idea,' he called as soon as they were in earshot.

Chris lined up next to Faye. 'Hello, gorgeous,' she said.

He raised his eyebrows at her. 'What's the matter? Can't stand the competition?'

'We'll see. You'll either fall off or get yourself assaulted dressed like that. I'm going to take it nice and slowly but I bet I'll be there before you.'

He looked at her patronisingly. 'I suppose you can always use your bus pass if you get tired.'

I shouted to get their attention. 'That's enough! We haven't even got to the start line and you're behaving badly already. Faye, you are old enough to know better. Chris, show more respect. Now, you know where to meet if we get lost, and if anybody feels tired or gets a puncture or anything, call me on the mobile. Oh, and drink loads of water. Don't get dehydrated. I'll try to keep somewhere in the middle of you. It's going to get crowded at Turner's Hill and Ditchling Beacon and only complete idiots try to ride those sections. I expect you to walk up them.' I looked at Chris. 'Except for you. I want to see you ride every inch of the way.'

ALCOHOL

Alcohol is a drug, but it's also the highest-calorie quick fix for stress, apart from over-eating. It's fast becoming our third major health hazard in the UK after heart disease and cancer. There are 70 calories in a glass of wine, it doesn't add anything to your diet nutritionally and it can even cause vitamin deficiencies.

Another problem with alcohol is that, being a depressant, it often stops you noticing how much you're eating.

It took forever to get through the start line. But eventually we were off. For the first few miles we stayed together, but gradually the younger ones pulled ahead. I wasn't worried. In spite of what I'd said, it was a relief not to have to watch Chris waving at everybody who wolf whistled him as he shot past them. I had to admit, he was extremely fit.

At one point I lost Faye completely and wasted quite a bit of time trying to find her. Eventually I gave up and pulled in for a snack. It was eleven o'clock by then and we'd been cycling for over two hours. I was in the queue at one of the roadside tea stands when she walked past me, a cup of tea in one hand and a huge slab of bread pudding in the other.

'Sorry, Pete I was desperate for a cup of tea so I went on ahead. I knew you'd catch up.'

When I'd got my drink and sandwich I went over to join her. 'How's it going, Faye? You'd better be drinking lots of water as well as that tea.'

'I am. And this is my breakfast, by the way. I was too nervous to eat when we set off. That's one of the things I changed since I've been under your influence. I still can't eat anything first thing, but I find that if I have something late morning as soon as I get hungry, I don't keep wanting to pick at bits in the afternoon like I used to.'

'So what do you do, take an early lunch break?'

'I can't do that, but I take something with me now. I used to skip breakfast and then I had to hang on till one o clock. But,' she paused and smiled at me, 'I've been working on that Personal Eating Plan. I couldn't have done it before because I didn't know myself well enough. I either didn't have a plan at all, or I tried to live by other people's. Now I know when I need to have food by me and when I'm likely to get hungry. It suits me to have a really early lunch, then something mid afternoon. And I don't eat as late in the evening as I used to. It wouldn't work for everybody but my body feels happy with it. Eating sensibly earlier in the day seems right. I even know now that some days I'm just not as hungry as others.' She licked her fingers. 'I used to think you had to eat the same amount regularly if you wanted to be healthy. Mind you, it feels really good to be as hungry as this. I can't remember the last time something tasted this wonderful.'

'The days you're feeling hungrier than usual there's usually a reason. Today it's obvious, but there will be other days when your body will have its reasons too. How's the ride going?'

'Sore bum, but that's about it. If I ever do this again I'm bringing a cushion like that man over there.'

'Think you'll make it the rest of the way?'

'No problem. How about you?'

ALCOHOL

Spend more on buying high quality and drink less of it.

Take your drink slowly. Wine with a meal isn't just for washing down the food.

Drink water with alcohol and don't drink on an empty stomach.

Never use alcohol to quench thirst. It's a diuretic.

If you drink spirits at home, think small pub measures.

Ask yourself, is there a healthier option, like wine or beer?

The fewer chemicals in your drink, the less harm it will do. Read the labels.

Be aware of how alcohol is making you feel and how much you have drunk.

Drink at your own pace, unless it's faster than everybody else's.

In fact I didn't really have time to think about whether I was tired or not. Keeping track of a group of fifty isn't easy in a crowd of thousands. As it was, I should have been paying more attention to the road. I was five miles from our meeting point just outside Brighton when I rode over the broken glass and about half a mile later when I realised I had a puncture. It took me twenty minutes to get back on the road again and by the time I got to the top of Ditchling Beacon it was an hour and a half since I'd seen any of the others. The relief when I caught sight of them, spread out over the South Downs in the sunshine was enormous. I got off the bike and walked over.

Ben stood up and moved his bike closer to the others to make space for me. 'What happened to you Pete?'

'I was trying to keep track of you all, then I got a puncture. Is everybody here?'

'More or less,' said Lewis. He was lying on the grass with his eyes closed, a can of sport drink in his hand.

Lisa was kneeling beside him, eating a cheese roll. She looked bright and enthusiastic. 'I'm starving. I told Lewis he needed to eat something substantial, a sandwich and a flapjack or something. But he just keeps drinking that luminous green stuff. Its not doing him any good.'

Lewis reached out and grabbed her wrist without opening his eyes. 'Listen, bossyboots, I used to live on sugar and caffeine before you came on the scene. I've nearly given it all up for you. I don't even drink much beer any more…'

Ben, who was sitting nearby, looked sceptical. 'That depends on what you call 'much'.' He waved a water bottle at Lewis. 'But Lisa has got it right. Water's just as good – I must have drunk two litres already this morning.'

Lisa smiled. 'Thank you Ben. Proved right again. Actually, apart from being thirsty the only problem I've had with this trip so far is my make-up running.'

'Mine isn't,' said Chris.

Lisa looked interested. 'How do you manage that?'

'Stage makeup. It stays on under spotlights and it stays on when you're exercising.'

I went and sat next to Lewis. 'Lisa's right. You need some complex carbohydrate. Those sport drinks are mostly sugar and water, they won't give you the staying power.'

He opened one eye. 'Not you as well. Alright, I'll go and get something. How much further have we got?'

'We're nearly there. Ten miles. You've done fifty already. And the last bit's all downhill.'

Whatever a man sows, that he will also reap.

Galatians VI v.vii

Jane stood up and counted. 'Everybody's here. How are you all? Any aches and pains, any problems? I can take a look now if anybody thinks they've strained something' We'd appointed her official masseuse to the Lighten Up team.

Everybody put their hands up and Jane shook her head at them. 'I can't do everybody so I assume that you're all able to continue.'

'We'll be brave,' said Faye. 'Getting back on that saddle's going to be the worst.'

Jane laughed. 'I ride a bike every day and even I'm feeling it. Listen up now, those of you who come to my Monday night circuit training. Tomorrow we are going to have a gentle relaxation session instead. I don't care how keen you are. Everybody will ache a bit tomorrow because none of us rides sixty miles regularly enough. And when you get home tonight I advise you that this is the time to go for the relaxing bath, the aromatherapy oils, and the lucky ones can ask their nearest and dearest to give them a massage. You're bodies have been amazing today. Be nice to them in return.'

Eventually everybody was ready and I got them back on their bikes with their team T-shirts. Chris put up a token objection that it didn't go with the rest of his outfit. 'You designed them,' I pointed out.

'Well don't put him in charge of the team colours next year,' said Faye. 'God knows what we'll end up wearing.'

"Oh no," I thought to myself, "they want to do this again."

Then the best bit happened. We were on the downhill run, keeping pretty much together with Brighton in sight, which wasn't easy with the number of bikes on the road. I was at the back when I heard a yell from the front of the pack. I thought I must have mis-heard. I overtook them all and got up to the front. 'What's happening?' At that moment I saw her. She'd obviously been waiting for us and came cycling in from a lay-by, laughing at the amazement on our faces. She looked tired, but very determined and she was wearing one of the T-shirts. We were all cheering as Mo took her place at the front of the group and crossed the line ahead of the rest of us.

In the chaos after the finishing line I felt a tug on my arm. I looked round. 'Go to the West Pier and head for the flag,' said Mo.

'What flag?' but she was gone.

When I eventually fought my way through the crowd and cycled slowly along the prom to the West Pier, I tried to spot a landmark. Like Chris. But the first thing I saw, was a bunch of balloons and a flag with 'Pete's Lighten Up Group'. As I chained up my bike and walked across the stones I wondered who'd carried them down. I hadn't noticed any of my team with balloons. A lot of them seemed to have got there faster than me, Chris included, and he'd taken the high heels off at last. Not surprisingly. It's difficult enough to walk across that beach at the best of times.

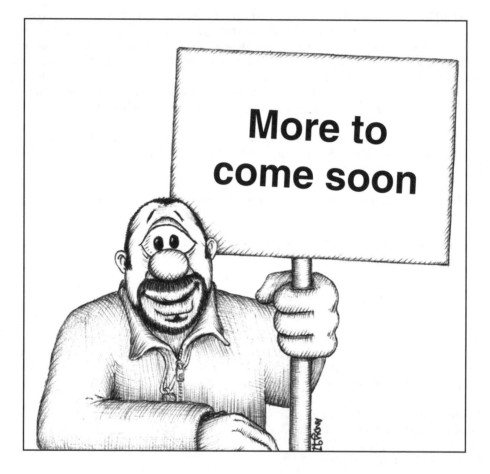

As I got closer, I realised there was a cloth spread out with food and cold boxes. The balloons were tied to an ice bucket. I heard a familiar voice. 'Surprise, surprise!' Eve was just getting to her feet, a bottle of champagne in her hand.

The others were right behind me. 'Did you all know about this?' I asked them.

'Nobody knew, except Mo and Faye until the very last minute,' Eve said. 'We thought of telling you and then we thought it would be fun to give you a surprise. What happened was, me and Faye went round to see Mo a couple of nights ago. It was obvious that none of the rest of you were going to sort her out so we thought it was time to tell her to pull herself together.'

Mo took up the story. 'I'd been thinking about joining in for a couple of weeks but I was still feeling pretty negative, then it got really close to the time and I looked at my bike and realised it needed a lot doing to it. I haven't ridden it for ages.'

Eve pointed across at the bike Mo had been riding. 'I lent her mine. I knew I wasn't going to make that distance. I might next year, but I wasn't going to push myself beyond my limits. Anyway, I've had almost as much exercise as you lot just carrying all this stuff from the van. My husband helped me load it up at home, but I was on my own when I got down here. And I must have parked two miles away at least. Mo did the catering by the way, I just did the driving!'

Mo looked at Eve in concern. 'I didn't push you into driving when you really wanted to come by bike, did I?'

'No, Love, don't start worrying about that. Of course you didn't. I'm not saying these have been the best weeks of my life. In fact I've had a couple of difficult days where I went off the rails and I didn't stick to my outcomes or anything else. And evenings when I totally veered off the Food Cake. But I've looked back and I've learned from them. I'm not running away from anything. Six months ago I couldn't have spent a morning in a van with a picnic for forty people. But I was just great today. I seem to have lost the knack of making myself feel really bad and I used to be so good at it.

'Oh, Pete, I have to tell you this.' Mo was handing round plates and glasses. She looked at me sideways. 'Thank you for those beliefs you wrote on the board. I felt so bad that night you came round I couldn't find any positive ones of my own. I adapted those ones you wrote on the board and I had them all installed by last Friday. Hard wired in. There was only one problem though.'

'What was that?'

'The cat nearly starved because I wouldn't let Lisa rub them off till I felt I could cope again. We always write the shopping lists up there and we can get takeaways, but he can't!'

Lewis leaned across to take a spoonful of rice salad. 'It did him the world of good. He's been getting out and about more. He's usually too busy eating or sleeping it off to force himself through the cat flap.'

REMINDERS

Eat when you are hungry

Use the Hunger Scale to find out how hungry you really are

Eat slowly so that you know when you are full

If you are triggered to eat for any reason other than hunger, do something else

Continue to incorporate exercise and activity into your daily life

Look to separate eating from other activities and enjoy it

Drink plenty of water throughout the day

Be positive about yourself and expect to learn from all your experiences

Mo picked up the bowl and passed it to me. 'Help yourself to some food. I promise you it's loaded with fibre and complex carbohydrates. In fact it's all very healthy, except the champagne of course – and we bought that out of our Fun Jars – since you said we had to use them for something frivolous.' She caught my eye. 'OK, I know it should have been something non-fattening as well, but this is a special occasion.'

'There's one thing I meant to ask you, Pete,' said Eve. 'Do we have to keep a food diary for the rest of our lives?'

'You can if you want to. But you'll probably find it doesn't turn out to be a food diary. You might want to write down your goals, achievements and ambitions, for example. They're nice to have around you in writing for those days when you feel a bit fed up or you lose sight of where you're going. Remember that research in America that said you're much more likely to achieve things you write down? Why don't you go home tonight and write in your diary that you cycled all the way to Brighton?'

'I'm hardly going to forget this, am I?' said Faye.

'But then, write down exactly how you felt about that achievement. How you feel while you're sitting here on the beach. We forget those good feelings. Get them down on paper. They can be very useful later on. Good memories on tap when you need them.'

At that moment someone in the distance caught my attention.

'What's the matter, Pete?'

'I was sure I saw Chris over there, but he's right here, isn't he? I saw him a moment ago.'

Mo laughed. 'The worry of organising this must have upset you more than we thought. Or maybe you weren't breathing deeply enough while you were pedalling. Just concentrate on holding this steady for a minute.' She bent over my glass and carefully filled it.

'Can we join you?'

I looked up again. And did a double take. Miriam was looming over me, high heels in one hand and the other holding her skirt together where it had split at the side. Her hairdo had collapsed but she was laughing.

Chris hopped over the stones and shook her by the hand. Fortunately she dropped the shoes.

They were wearing identical outfits – apart from the T-shirts – but Chris's makeup had survived intact. I knew that wig of his reminded me of someone.

Realisation was starting to dawn on me. 'Alright, what's been going on?'

REMINDERS

Remember there is no such thing as failure, only feedback

Eat a balanced diet with a variety of food from different food groups

Eat fresh, natural produce wherever possible

Be patient and give yourself plenty of credit as you develop new patterns

Be lucky and enjoy your life

Remember, the most important thing is to have focus and point in the right direction. This way you'll always know where you're going

The right way

'Well,' said Eve, producing a notebook. 'Miriam and Chris got together and decided we could raise much more money if we pooled our resources and did some sort of stunt. We were going to tell you and then we decided to make it a surprise. I was really worried about you seeing it in the local paper though.'

Jane came over. 'I had to hide the office copy for the last three weeks.'

'I thought they'd just stopped delivering it to the club. So, tell me the rest of it.'

'How do you know there's any more to tell?'

'You've got it written all over your faces. First of all, how much did you raise for charity?'

'Nearly a thousand.'

'So who wins the bet?' asked Faye.

'Well, Chris was here first, wasn't he?' said Eve. 'According to this,' she consulted her notebook, '25 people bet on Chris and 37 on Miriam.'

There was a howl of rage from Chris. 'You mean people actually put money on her instead of me? Let me see that book.'

'Certainly not,' Eve snatched it away from him. 'You obviously don't inspire confidence in everybody. Anyway, what are you complaining about? You got here first so your honour's satisfied.

Miriam lay down on the stones and stretched out in the sun. 'Make the most of it, Chris. Next year, it won't be so easy. I'm going into training. I haven't had so much fun in ages. Reminds me of my dancing days, putting on a show. I haven't given a thought to what my group have been eating. She opened her eyes and sat up. 'By the way, Pete, what is the difference that makes the difference?'

'It's different for everybody. But you probably just summed it up for you.' I told her. 'There are two important things to remember, how good you feel and how slim you are. It's just a question of getting them in the right order. And only you know how to do that.'

Lighten Up

46 Staines Road
Twickenham
Twickenham TW2 5AH

Tel: 020 8241 2323
Fax: 020 8241 2268
E-mail: info@lightenup.co.uk

Or visit our website:
www.lightenup.co.uk

Workshops and Courses
Eight-week evening courses (two hours a week, usually on Monday nights) are running in North and South London alternately throughout the year.

One-day workshops, from 10.00am to 5.00pm, one Saturday or Sunday each month, in North or South London.

Workshops outside London
Call us for details.

Audio Tapes
Pete Cohen's first tape, on which he talks you through his techniques, is now available by mail order from the above address at £9.99 and £1.50 postage and packing.

TV, Radio, Magazines and Newspapers
Pete writes regularly for some magazines and appears regularly in all the media. Watch out for him!

Doing it with Pete
The sequel to *Slimming With Pete* takes you step by step through the same Lighten Up weight loss programme, so that you can uncover for yourself the slimmer, fitter, healthier 'blueprint' of the real you. This Lighten Up slimming fun book guides you through each exercise in a practical, easy-to-follow style that is readable and entertaining. It is available from bookshops as well as by mail order at £12.99 and £2.50 postage and packing.

Let us know what you think:
We would love to hear from you. Please contact Maria or Judith by mail, phone, fax or e-mail and let us have your feedback.

Other titles from

Crown House Publishing
www.crownhouse.co.uk

Doing it with Pete
The Lighten Up Slimming Fun Book
Pete Cohen & Judith Verity

The sequel to the bestselling *Slimming With Pete*. While its hugely popular predecessor treated us to the fascinating story of the first Lighten Up group, this highly readable manual gets straight down to business, communicating in a crystal-clear manner the exact techniques used in Pete's famous Lighten Up programme. It appeals for two reasons. First, it is an easy-to-handle book with many cartoon illustrations and clear, focused blocks of text. It is, simply, a pleasure to use and peruse. Second, it offers the most enjoyable and comprehensive way to "get into" the Lighten Up programme. The exercises are presented separately and lucidly, and are arranged to form a complete and easy-to-follow scheme for slimming. For the first time this programme is available in the form of a completely user-oriented workbook – a guide to slimming using Pete's techniques.

PAPERBACK   256 PAGES   ISBN: 1899836195

Emotionally Intelligent Living
Geetu Orme

Most people have probably heard of Emotional Intelligence (EI) already. In recent years it has been pondered, theorised and explained in exhaustive scientific detail, prominently profiled in the press and on the Internet. EI has proven its existence and proclaimed itself to the world. Now it is time to *act* upon its remarkable conclusions.

Enter *Emotionally Intelligent Living*. This is not a book to read, it is a book to *do* – an EI tool that applies the theory to life. If the whole EI phenomenon has passed you by, don't worry – this book begins with a practical summary of what EI is, explaining it in the clearest terms that require no previous knowledge of psychology. Immediately, it makes EI relevant to everyday reality, presenting case studies of Emotionally Intelligent people, and providing an essential preliminary exercise that allows you to *measure your own Emotional Quotient (EQ)*.

Now comes the good news: EI *can* be learnt, and your EQ *can* be increased. This book contains a unique programme of emotional improvement that will revolutionise your ability to use your emotions effectively. Targeting the most practical benefits of EI, *Emotionally Intelligent Living* systematically implements its insights in the following areas of life:

▲ business	▲ success
▲ friendships	▲ teams
▲ careers	▲ families
▲ leadership	▲ partner relationships

Designed to be as eminently easy-to-use and enjoyable to peruse as possible, *Emotionally Intelligent Living* serves as an excellent EI resource with its inclusion of an extensive list of worldwide EQ resources (including websites), and the most up-to-date EI assessment techniques. Packed with brilliant strategies for emotional management, and inspirational ideas for focusing your feelings, it offers you the very best methods for putting the theory into practice and living an emotionally intelligent life.

PAPERBACK   220 PAGES   ISBN: 1899836470

Socialising For Success
The NLP Guide to Perfecting Your Social Skills
Clare Walker

Have you ever wished that you could enjoy socialising at work? Instead of being a chore to be endured, have you dreamed that the endless small talk over lunch could be turned into a genuinely interesting event? Or maybe you've always wondered how someone in your department managed to gain their promotion so young, when you know far more than they do about the subject, and yet they are always talking, talking, talking. And succeeding. How do they do it?

This books tells you *exactly* how. *Socialising For Success* presents you with NLP-based techniques that will enable you to approach workplace and business socialising with genuine confidence. Your increasing enjoyment of these occasions *and* your colleagues will create the conditions in which interesting opportunities can arise for you. The net benefit will be a more rapid career advancement!

At the core of this book lies the observation that skills are simply *a combination of particular behaviours, strategies, thought patterns and beliefs*. Taking you step-by-step through the process of creating new, socially successful skills, *Socialising For Success* teaches you:

- ▲ how to build a belief structure that supports successful socialising
- ▲ how to create a motivating vision of successful socialising
- ▲ communication strategies you can depend upon
- ▲ techniques that will enable you to perform effortlessly at every social event
- ▲ follow-up strategies that turn socialising into an ongoing enjoyment of life.

PAPERBACK   240 PAGES   ISBN: 189983625X

Warriors, Settlers & Nomads
Terence Watts

Are you a Warrior? Are you a Settler? Are you a Nomad?

Identifying your predominant personality-type changes the way you approach life. If you know *yourself* – and, equally important, if you understand *other* people – you can confidently tackle your career and your personal relationships knowing exactly where you are coming from – *and* what everyone else is seeking.

Warriors, Settlers & Nomads presents a revolutionary framework with which to comprehend your own needs, and the needs of others. Based upon the concept of evolutionary psychology, it reveals the determinants at the core of our characters – those very skills and psychological attitudes that we have inherited from our ancestors. Teaching us how we have all retained features of three ancient tribes – the *Warriors*, the *Settlers*, and the *Nomads* – this book guides us through revealing personality tests and detailed descriptions of each tribe trait, allowing us to identify our specific type – the basic mould from which we are produced – and to appreciate the wisdoms and strengths that up to now have lain dormant inside us.

A guide to self-discovery and self-liberation, *Warriors, Settlers & Nomads* utilises powerful hypnosis and visualisation techniques in a programme designed to release our hidden potential. A fascinating and revelatory read, it provides unique personal growth strategies that enable us to discover *who we really are*.

PAPERBACK   252 PAGES   ISBN: 1899836489

Orders to:

The Anglo American Book Company Ltd.
Crown Buildings,
Bancyfelin, Carmarthen,
Wales,
SA33 5ND
UK
www.anglo-american.co.uk

Tel: 01267 211880/211886
(Lines open 9am – 5.30pm Mon – Fri)
Fax: 01267 211882
E-mail: books@anglo-american.co.uk

Or visit the
Crown House Publishing Website at:
www.crownhouse.co.uk